Psychosocial Interventions in End-of-Life Care

T0271992

The concept of a "good death" has been hotly debated in medical circles for decades. This volume delves into the possibility and desirability of a "good death" by presenting the psychosocial measures of care as a crucial component, such as religion, existentialism, hope and meaning-making. The volume also focuses on oncologic psychiatry and the influence of technology as a means to alleviate pain and suffering, and potentially provide relief to those at the end of life. Such initiatives are aimed at diminishing pain and are socially bolstering and emotionally comforting to ensure a peaceful closure with life as opposed to a battle waged.

Utilizing the most recent information from medical journals and books to present the latest on healthcare and dying today, this volume crosses the boundaries of thanatology, psychology, religion, spirituality, medical ethics and public health.

Peggy Sturman Gordon received her second Master's degree in Thanatology from Brooklyn College, USA. In addition she is a trained art and horticultural therapist and has worked with the geriatric population for more than a decade.

Research in Death Studies

Books in This Series:

Psychosocial Interventions in End-of-Life Care
The Hope for a "Good Death"
Peggy Sturman Gordon

Psychosocial Interventions in End-of-Life Care

The Hope for a "Good Death"

Peggy Sturman Gordon

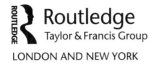

Routledge
Taylor & Francis Group

LONDON AND NEW YORK

First published 2016 by Routledge

2 Park Square, Milton Park, Abingdon, Oxon OX14 4RN
711 Third Avenue, New York, NY 10017, USA

Routledge is an imprint of the Taylor & Francis Group,
an informa business

First issued in paperback 2017

Library of Congress Cataloguing-in-Publication Data
Gordon, Peggy Sturman.
Psychosocial interventions in end-of-life care : the hope for a good death / by
   Peggy Sturman Gordon.
      pages cm
   Includes bibliographical references.
   1. Terminal care—Psychological aspects.   2. Terminal care—Social
aspects.   3. Terminally ill—Care.   I. Title.
   R726.8.G687 2016
   616.02'9—dc23   2015030527

ISBN: 978-1-138-79759-8 (hbk)
ISBN: 978-1-138-08609-8 (pbk)

Typeset in Sabon
by Apex CoVantage, LLC

Contents

Figures

Series Editor Introduction

Peggy Sturman Gordon's book offers a comprehensive synthesis about contemporary encounters with the end of life. She takes the story beyond North America and brings in an international perspective, including European, Asian, and Australian points of view on the end of life. She offers in one volume a wide-ranging look at efforts by pioneers in the hospice movement and more recently in palliative medicine to make a good death both a possibility for terminally ill persons and a norm for medical practitioners. She underscores that dying, as part of living, is a multidimensional experience, and thus that achieving a good death requires attention to the holistic realities whereby human beings face their possibilities and make their choices. We are pleased to offer *Psychosocial Interventions in End-of-Life Care: The Hope for a "Good Death"* as the initial volume in this new monograph series, *Research in Death Studies*.

The dying trajectories and principal causes of death in developed countries have changed dramatically over the past century. Whereas a typical dying trajectory in the early 20th century was sudden and unexpected death due to a fatal, infectious disease or accident, the process of dying has become principally a lingering, drawn-out trajectory involving a series of chronic, debilitating conditions. A major factor that has produced these changes in dying trajectories and causes of death is the triumph of the biomedical model and its fundamental goal to maintain life at all costs. Other influences have come from advances in the production and protection of food, success in insuring clean water, architectural and engineering triumphs (buildings with better heating and cooling, for instance), and public health campaigns educating communities about healthy and unhealthy behaviors.

The triumph of the biomedical model is no doubt due to its success in producing new knowledge and in overcoming previously fatal diseases. The biomedical model has gained widespread cultural acceptance in developed countries. On the whole, most persons in developed countries in the 21st century view life, health, disease, and death from within the assumptive world of the biomedical model.

A clear upshot of the success of the biomedical model is that large numbers of individuals live significantly beyond their 60s and develop the many infirmities endemic to aging bodies and minds. Associated with many progressive infirmities is the presence of functional limitation, such as difficulty walking, stooping, or swallowing. For example, of the nearly 313 million persons in the USA, 14% (nearly 44 million) have both chronic, debilitating conditions and functional limitations, and this 14% of the population accrues over 56% of all health care costs incurred in the USA. These figures will only increase as the aging population continues to grow. In many cases, these persons form a new societal phenomenon, the "frail elderly."

What is of considerable concern is when life-prolonging technologies produce a continuation of life bereft of quality. Some commentators, in fact, refer to a prolongation of dying, rather than a continuation of living, when medical interventions keep persons alive but helpless, incontinent, lacking dignity, connected to all sorts of instruments, and in pain.

The realities that many persons die in a lingering, pain-filled trajectory filled with intrusive medical procedures—procedures that extend length of life but diminish quality of life—have inspired efforts to allow terminally ill persons to die a good death. Many persons at the end-of-life face prospects that do not match individual preferences about dying. Whereas the desires are for a painless death in familiar surroundings with the presence of loved ones, the stark reality is that most persons die in institutionalized settings, in pain, hooked up to medical machinery, and surrounded by strangers. Not wishing to be victimized by a medical approach that chooses to keep persons alive at all costs, people have sought alternatives that keep intact their autonomy and self-determination in the face of imminent death. People have sought options that increase the possibility of dying a good death.

David E. Balk
Series Editor
August 2015

Introduction

> . . . death has a bad reputation. Words like awful and catastrophic are practically synonymous with death. Good and death seem oxymoronic, incompatible, mutually exclusive. Given this, what then can it mean to speak of a good death? Are some deaths better than others? Can one plan to improve on one's death?
>
> (Shneidman, 2007, p. 245)

Good Death, Good Enough Death, Decent Death, Acceptable Death, Appropriate Death, Purposeful Death, Aware Death, Respectful Death, Soulless Death, Sudden Death, Patient Centered Death, Well-Managed Death, Peaceful Death, Smooth Death, Dignified Death, Consistent Death, Rational Death, Gentle Death, Timely Death, Postmodern Death, Natural Death, Idealized Death, Healthy Death, Romantic Death, Correct Death, Brave Death, Self-Chosen Death, Self-Actualized Death, Happy Death, Bad Death . . .

Each of the above modifiers of death has been mentioned by one or more writers who have studied and written about death. The concept of a good death bears a diversity of meanings from a range of theoretical disciplines. Thanatologists, social anthropologists, sociologists, physicians, nurses, theologians, psychologists, and psychiatrists have all written on the topic and agree on the most basic hallmarks: appropriate preparations, symptom control, social support, and spiritual peace. The good death concept focuses on the core of the dying experience and death event that involves the presence of physical symptoms, spiritual/existential concerns, family and community support, life satisfaction, and feelings of loss and grief (Granda-Cameron & Houldin, 2012).

Death is not a disease or an illness. "Death is inevitable, a fact of nature, a human universal. Death is the greatest democracy of all" (Feifel, 1977, p. 5). "Death is inexorable" (Weisman, 1972, 1974, p. 12). "Death is the defining event of old age" (Kearl, 1996, p. 336). "Death is nonbeing . . . the antithesis of life" (Byock, 2002, p. 279). ". . . death is natural and necessary and inextricably tied to life. To live is to be mortal; death is the necessary price of life. . . . When we 'buy' life we 'buy' death (Leon Kass, in Callahan, 1977, p. 35).

However, Weisman contended that the most commonly held view of death is that it is evil, the ultimate catastrophe (1972; 1974, p. 139). If death is the obverse of birth, a part of living, lifestyle vs. death-style, why does life's natural outcome bear a taboo? Is it possible to salvage a good death from amongst the malevolent ruins of evil?

Modern humans have faced death more directly and frequently than ever before, due to media and communications that cross oceans, instead of limiting the world to one's immediate vicinity (Weisman, 1974). Still, humans are not accustomed to death. In fact, humans are frightened to death about death (Weisman, 1972). Many people feel that death is a regrettable necessity, and still harbor a primitive belief that suitable negotiation is possible so that death might not be compulsory. The realm of death has been forbidden and carries a taboo, from which we are protected by rituals and rites, and by those we choose to conduct them. Death bears elements of both the sacred and the sinister such that anyone associated with it acquires something of its taboo and special awe. These people, such as physicians or clergy, are educated to intercede in our behalf, to forestall death or, if they cannot, to relieve our anguish (Weisman, 1972). Because healthcare professionals are those most in contact with the sick and dying, it is they who develop sufficient experience with death and dying. Therefore, one would suppose that it is they who must provide for the possibility of a good death.

Even though humans recognize death as universal, we cannot imagine our own death: other people die, personal death has no reality. Death, when it comes, therefore takes us by surprise and finds us in bewilderment and denial. Ernest Becker, whose book, *The Denial of Death* (1973), won a Pulitzer Prize for his thesis that an innate terror of death exists in all of us, bearing the beneficent effect of being the mainspring of all human cultures and creativity. Becker's exploration of heroism holds that humans strive to the heroic "in order to earn a feeling of primary value . . . of ultimate usefulness to creation, of unshakable meaning. . . . The hope and belief is that the things that man creates in society are of lasting worth and meaning, that they outshine the death and decay . . ." (Becker, 1973, p. 5). Becker's more contemporary followers, Pyszczynski, Greenberg, and Solomon (1999) empirically tested some of Becker's claims and advanced the terror management theory: that our ancestor's discovery of their mortality evolved to help us manage the anxiety generated by that discovery. Weisman (1972) put forth another perspective about fear of death from a psychological viewpoint, that "death is a universal phobia to be avoided" (p. 13), a reflection of man's "helplessness" (p. 15).

Perhaps what is missing is a positive ideal of a good death rather than the avoidance of healthcare problems and bad interventions. However, society today seems to accept as true that death is optional, that "aging and death need not be a part of one's life so long as one exercises, has regular check-ups and eats healthfully" (Callahan, 2009, p. 106). We are led to this belief by the prodigious accomplishments of technology that now prevent disease or cure us of it, thereby prolonging our lives. How we look at death and dying coexists with a denial of death headlined by the desire for youth and the quest for longevity that remains the "primary standard for evaluating healthcare systems" (Emanuel & Emanuel, 1998, p. 21). This healthcare paradox presents as an "increasing concern about death and dying, tremendous technical capacities to relieve symptoms and improve health outcomes, and the persistent suffering of dying patients, all combined with the continued denial of death" (p. 21).

Is a good death one wherein a terminally ill patient faces: dying a prolonged death while undergoing aggressive, unwanted treatment, frequently on life support systems, in an acute care hospital, often with severe pain and fatigue, dyspnea, and dysphoria (Lynn et al., 1997)? In fact individuals regularly have died under such circumstances, either when alternatives were not immediately controllable or by electing to die in such a way, by insisting that the physician do "everything". What does everything look like and is it preferable?

Is a good death feasible, practicable, achievable, viable, desirable, or, for that matter, even considered at all? And, if so, is death thought of in terms of quality, value, or worth? In terms of pleasure, contentment, or happiness? Does a good death exist? If so, what makes for a good death, in contrast to one filled with anguish and despair? The answer, seemingly, is simple, but in actuality the response to these questions is multi-faceted, complex, and fluid. The very idea of a good death is ambiguous, context-dependent, the subject of diverse cultural, sub-cultural, and individual meanings, beset with tensions and paradox (Masson, 2002).

Whereas death is a natural event, it has traditionally been viewed as the enemy of the medical profession, its failure: "Death is to the doctor the last enemy, the ultimate defeat of his dedication to health and life" (Saclier, 1976, p. 5). The experience encountered by today's adults as they face mortality has been shaped by new medical, demographic, and cultural trends. More of us live longer and die later from chronic, rather than acute diseases; our lives are protected by powerful medications and upheld by machines designed to prolong life, albeit with dubious quality. Such progress in diagnosing and prolonging the survival of patients with advanced disease has created a "new experience of dying, one dominated by a prolonged, indeterminate state of living/dying, which can last for years" (Nissim et al., 2012, p. 378). Further, Green (2008) observed that today's baby boomers, "the most catered-to generation in American history" (p. 3), are facing the mortality of their elderly parents and beginning to recognize their own temporal limitations. They face a less-hidden, less-whispered about death—a *death* not a *passing*—that has evolved to be less religious and more individualized. Religion has become marginalized and replaced by psychology practitioners.

In the medical model of death today, dying is about heroic struggle and control, about attempting to manage the timing and manner of our exit: "The determination to be in control, to win small, temporary victories along the way, and to be in charge up to the last drives this model" (Green, 2008, p. 17). Controlling the dying process includes both the desire to "lengthen the period of meaningful living by maximizing treatment options and to avoid a painful, lingering death by considering suicide as an exit plan" (Nissim et al., 2012, p. 369). However, obtaining a good death challenges even the most careful planning.

Thus, is modern medicine contributing to achievement of a good death and to what extent? For all our quantifying, qualifying, experimenting and measuring, what have we learned? The information presented in this book looks at the variables that such an achievement potentially depends on: the much-investigated, objective factors such as the degree of symptomatic distress, the cause and location of the death, the quality of end of life care, the nature of family and other social support, and the personal qualities of the patient (Hales et al., 2010; Emanuel & Emanuel, 1998; Singer et al., 1999). While the evaluation of a death is inherently subjectively determined, such a judgment is influenced by numerous physical and psychosocial factors when humans come to die—when cells die off and body systems fail. How does one resolve such a crisis? How do those patients facing imminent death manage to live with this knowledge? Does denial work? Can the search for meaning and hope be called upon? Is there a will to live?

The information presented in this book attempts to clarify the concept of the good death and its presentation in scholarly writing, while exploring the ways in which attaining one may be approached, if not ensured. As one of the ways to attain a good death is implementing psychosocial interventions that may serve to improve the end of life, psychosocial concepts will also be investigated. The material focuses on the populations of North America, Western Europe, Asia, and Australia and on the particular issues faced by the elderly with a life-limiting illness or terminal condition who are approaching death. The understanding and perceptions of death and dying differ even within developed countries where populations are varied by culture, education, socioeconomic status and, of course, by fear and misinformation.

A brief history of death traditions in Western civilization provides the context of the subject, and continues to the advent of modern ideas of death awareness that began after World War II. Thereafter, in attempting to characterize the concept of a good death, research pertaining to a good death is presented specifically within the subject areas of public policy, the delivery of end-of-life care and its resulting quality of death and dying, and the role of hospice and palliative care. Psychosocial paradigms and potential interventions that have been shown to improve the quality of life as death approaches are then introduced: the roles of dignity, spirituality and religion, hope and meaning making. Finally, the concept of the good death as it has been discussed over the years will be presented and summarized.

CITATIONS: INTRODUCTION

Becker, E. (1973). *The denial of death*. New York: The Free Press/A Division of Macmillan Publishing.

Byock, I. (2002). The meaning and value of death. *Journal of Palliative Medicine, 5*(2), 279–289.

Callahan, D. (1977). On defining a "natural death." *The Hastings Center Report, 7*(3), 32–37.

Callahan, D. (2009). Death, mourning, and medical progress. *Perspectives in Biology and Medicine, 52*(1), 103–115. http://doi.org/10.1353/pbm.0.0067.

Emanuel, E. J., & Emanuel, L. L. (1998). The promise of a good death. *Lancet, 351* (Suppl. II), SII21–SII29. Retrieved from www.ncbi.nlm.nih.gov/pubmed/9606363.

Feifel, H. (1977). Death in contemporary America. In H. Feifel (Ed.) *New meanings of death* (pp. 3–12). New York: McGraw Hill & Co.

Granda-Cameron, C., & Houldin, A. (2012). Concept analysis of good death in terminally ill patients. *The American Journal of Hospice & Palliative Care, 29*(8), 632–639. http://doi.org/10.1177/1049909111434976.

Green, J. W. (2008). *Beyond the good death: The anthropology of modern dying.* Philadelphia, PA: University of Pennsylvania Press.

Hales, S., Zimmermann, C., & Rodin, G. (2010). The quality of dying and death: A systematic review of measures. *Journal of Palliative Medicine, 24*(2), 127–144. http://doi.org/10.1177/0269216309351783.

Kearl, M. C. (1996). Dying well: The unspoken dimension of aging well. *American Behavioral Scientist, 39*(3), 336–360. http://doi.org/10.1177/00027642960390 03009.

Lynn, J., Teno, J. M., Phillips, R. S., Wu, A. W., Desbiens, N., Harrold, J., . . . Investigators, S. (1997). Perceptions by family members of the dying experience of older and seriously ill patients. *Annals of Internal Medicine, 126*(2), 97–106.

Masson, J. D. (2002). Non-professional perceptions of "good death": A study of the views of hospice care patients and relatives of deceased hospice care patients. *Mortality, 7*(2), 191–209. http://doi.org/10.1080/1357627022013629.

Nissim, R., Rennie, D., Fleming, S., Hales, S., Gagliese, L., & Rodin, G. (2012). Goals set in the land of the living/dying: A longitudinal study of patients living with advanced cancer. *Death Studies, 36*(4), 360–390. Retrieved from www.ncbi. nlm.nih.gov/pubmed/24567991.

Pyszczynski, T., Greenberg, J., & Solomon, S. (1999). A dual-process model of defense against conscious and unconscious death-related thoughts: An extension of terror management theory, *Psychological Review, 106*(4), 835–845.

Saclier, A. L. (1976). Good death. *Australian and New Zealand Journal of Psychiatry, 10*(1), 3–6. http://doi.org/10.3109/00048677609159478.

Shneidman, E. (2007). Criteria for a good death. *Suicide & Life-Threatening Behavior, 37*(3), 245–247. http://doi.org/10.1521/suli.2007.37.3.245.

Singer, P. A., Martin, D. K., Kelner, M. (1999). Quality end-of-life care: Patient's perspectives. *JAMA, 281*(2), 163–168.

Weisman, A. D. (1972). *On dying and denying*. New York: Behavioral Publications.

Weisman, A. D. (1974). *The realization of death*. New York & London: Jason Aronson Inc.

Part I
Aspects of Death and Dying

1   Western Attitudes to Death

A good death was more the norm prior to the explosion of technology in the 20th century, which fractured, not only atoms, but also families, neighborhoods, extended families, and communities. Where before an entire community routinely participated in the rituals of preparing a body for burial, in wakes and funerals, death today has been excommunicated from society and become a mystery to our contemporary population, hidden away in dark, cold basements.

1.1 HISTORIES OF DEATH: ARIÈS AND KELLEHEAR

> In the past few decades, medical science has rendered obsolete centuries of experience, tradition, and language about our mortality and created a new difficulty for mankind: how to die.
>
> (Atul Gawande, 2014, p. 158)

Two major views of the history of death and dying from ancient times to the social responsibilities of end-of-life care today were written by British sociologist Allan Kellehear and by the French social historian Philippe Ariès. Kellehear's *A Social History of Dying* (2007) presents a major review of the human and clinical sciences literature about human dying, an historical approach that places recent dying and death in broader historical, medical, and global context. Ariès initially wrote *Western Attitudes Toward Death: From the Middle Ages to the Present* (1974) as a series of lectures delivered at Johns Hopkins and in 1984 incorporated it into the book *The Hour of Our Death*. Ariès presented the development of Western attitudes to death in terms of four stages of historical development: the Tamed Death, One's Own Death, Thy Death, and Forbidden Death, which roughly match up with Kellehear's specification of eras in the history of death.

Kellehear began his historical account of death and dying in the Pastoral Age, the period he designated as occurring approximately between the Stone Age and the 15th century. Early on, death and dying came very suddenly and humans in this prehistoric era had no way to prepare for it. Evident from cave drawings of burial rites, humans gradually became personally aware of danger and began to inquire about life after death, preparing for an otherworld journey. Kellehear thereby identified one of the most important aspects of death which began in the Stone Age, that of its *anticipation*. The dying experience became a post death activity that was dependent upon the beliefs and behaviors of the survivors (Kellehear, 2007, pp. 27–9). The awareness of mortal illness led to exploration of ways to prevent mortality that resulted in the prehistoric suggestions of healing and sorcery, and eventually, centuries later, to biomedical technology and pharmacology (p. 49). Self-awareness of oncoming death, then, became the first feature of a good death (p. 87) that began to be recognized after World War II, to be studied by Glaser and Strauss and to become an indicator of positive psychosocial well-being.

The experience of death in the later Pastoral Age differed by virtue of the dying experience being predictable and anticipated, caused by infectious diseases that led to a gradual dying process and allowing the peasant or farmer to participate in his or her death. Such a death, wherein the dying person was able to prepare for his death with the assistance of his family, friends, and his community, was a good death, the result of a life well lived (Kellehear, 2007). This good death of peasants and farmers evolved as the industrial revolution and warfare began to transform society and healthcare.

Ariès's first period of death, Tamed Death, began in traditional peasant societies beginning in the early Middle Ages and lasted until about the 10th century. Then, as also described by Kellehear, a dying person knew and accepted that death was near and acted as the master of ceremonies over his or her own approaching death. The dying person presided over his or her last days, making farewells and seeking pardons, essentially repeating the rituals that he or she had witnessed as a younger person. Such rituals of dying and death, a public event that included the entire community, served as a public confirmation of humanity against an indifferent, callous Nature. These rituals were important, practiced ceremoniously, and conducted openly and freely, because death was known but not feared yet.

Ariès distinguished a change in death attitudes in the later Middle Ages, around AD 1000, wherein greater emphasis was placed on the significance of the moment of death and on the art of dying. Ariès referenced the pictorial art of the time, *Ars Moriendi*, which depicted various death scenes, such as the last judgment or scenes taking place in the bedchamber of the dying. Ariès called this historical stage of dying One's Own Death. The old collective rites of passage were still conducted, but with a new consciousness of the significance of the dying person as an individual (Boyd, 1977).

Ariès observed still another shift that began around the 16th century and is shown in the pictorial art as the Dance of Death, picturing death raping the living. Ariès saw this as a departure from the natural order, a violent disruption of daily life as it heretofore had been. The family of the dying person was then expected to do more, to take over the responsibility for the rituals of death from the dying person. The family was required to show and feel grief, eventually evolving into the hysterical mourning of the 19th century. By the advent of the 17th century, Thy Death, the understanding that such a death is one which happened to another, became emotionally exhausting to those who were charged with assuming the responsibility for the conduct of the death and of responding to it with feeling. As the family attempted to spare the dying person an undue ordeal, they also sought to spare themselves by avoiding strong emotion in the presence of death. This is Ariès's notion of the Forbidden Death, an attitude to death that sought to conceal its reality.

Ariès characterized the Wild Death, wherein no one had the right to become emotional except in private, secretly, because overt sorrow inspired repugnance rather than pity; such evident sorrow was considered too morbid and was a sign of mental instability or of bad manners. Within the family, one hesitated to show emotion for fear of upsetting the children (Ariès, 1974). To make this point, Ariès referred to the work of sociologist Geoffrey Gorer, as showing how, in the 20th century, the taboo of death replaced that of sex as the principal forbidden subject—something to withhold from the children: "Death has become more and more unmentionable as a *natural process*" (Gorer, 1955, p. 50).

By the 19th century, developments in the biological sciences revealed the relationship between disease symptoms and internal organs. Next, death came to be understood as arising from diseases or anomalies within the body. Death was made visible to the doctor, who tended to the patient and displaced religion and priests as the main attendants at the deathbed (Kaufman & Morgan, 2005). Death became an aspect of life. At that point, urban elites became prone to the degenerative diseases of aging, heart disease, and cancer, which engendered the management of complex economic, medical, and legal issues.

By the 20th century, the Forbidden Death had evolved into denial of the reality of death by ceding responsibilities to the hospital, where death took place quietly with the individual often under sedation and perhaps not even realizing what is occurring as he was surrounded by professionals (Boyd, 1977). Thus is achieved the "acceptable style of living while dying" (Ariès, 1974, p. 89). Ariès represents this modern death as the Wild Death, an inhumane and solitary way of dying, wherein both the family and dying person are outsiders. The doctor and hospital team are

> the masters of death . . . who try to obtain from their patient an acceptable style of living while dying. . . . An acceptable death is a death which can be accepted or tolerated by the survivors. It has its antithesis: the embarrassingly graceless dying, which embarrasses the survivors because it causes too strong an emotion to burst forth; and emotions must be avoided both in the hospital and everywhere in society.
>
> (Ariès, 1974, p. 89)

The rise of the city, accompanying the advent of the industrial revolution, produced a change in social relations: where pastoral societies were close-knit and community-oriented, urban societies "occurred in a context of mass population" (Kellehear, 2007, p. 147). Anonymity became a major cultural phenomenon in cities that contained a large range of communities. Mass migration combined with occupational diversification to place additional pressure on personal abilities to negotiate the day-to-day meanings and social and economic transactions. These sorts of transactions altered the nature of the good death and gave birth to the concept of what Kellehear called the Well-Managed Death. The awareness of dying was a major factor in both the good death and the well-managed death, but the well-managed death required confirmation by specialized others, such as medical professionals, who were able to manage the final tasks of the exit.

Death and dying became increasingly hidden during the course of the 20th century. The accustomed natural death "evolved from being respected to being unnatural and shameful, from being the culmination of a life to an unwanted interruption of existence" (Kearl, 1996, p. 338). Death began to be denied in order to avoid its unpleasantness while families usurped their loved one's autonomy in an effort to shield them, thereby undermining the ability to die well.

1.2 THE RISE OF THE INSTITUTIONAL CARE OF THE DYING

Kellehear made an important distinction between dying and death, particularly in today's modern world. Today, deaths occur in institutional settings, while " 'dying'—as a shared set of overt social exchanges between dying individuals and those who care for them—is increasingly unrecognised . . . has become . . . severed from its earlier biological, psychological and interpersonal moorings" (Kellehear, 2007, p. 253). Nowhere was this more evident than in the medical settings of hospitals where the thrust of managing death came to be controlled through institutionalization, medicalization, and bureaucratization. The organization of work by the hospital staff assumed greater importance than that of the dying individuals in their care. The lives of dying people in hospital were tightly controlled and became meaningless, isolated, and powerless, and devoid of autonomy (Hart et al., 1998). Social processes and events of the past, as noted by Ariès (1981), "were once spoken of and conducted more openly and freely, and those who were dying and grieving were far less isolated" (p. 67). The routinization of managing death contributed to the eventual establishment and success of hospice.

In the 1960s, sociologists joined the psychologists in studying death and dying within hospitals. Glaser and Strauss actually spent time in hospitals and published two books that contributed some important concepts about the dying process. In *Awareness of Dying* (1965) they documented what dying people knew or suspected about their impending death and the four awareness contexts and their influence on the dying process (see page xx). In their 1968 book, *Time for Dying*, Glaser and Strauss identified the dying trajectory, an objective picture of the good or appropriate death that was marked by hospital staffs' negotiation and management of critical events as the patient's status changed in progression towards death (Hart et al., 1998; Doka, 2007, p. 20). Subjectively, when professionals were confronted by a patient, Glaser and Strauss noted "fairly rapid estimations" about whether or not and how that individual might die (Corr et al., 1999, p. 244). Professionals organize their work and ill persons are treated in different ways on the basis of these estimates, such as bed assignment or use of more or less aggressive intervention. The importance of dying trajectories may then involve two elements of the same patient: "the disease processes internal to ill persons and important elements of assessment, communication, and interaction between dying persons and their care providers" (p. 244). Deaths which occur in an untimely manner present certain difficulties for the routinization and bureaucratization of staff and families.

David Sudnow was an ethnologist who studied the social organization of the modern hospital, that major setting of dying in our society (Sudnow, 1967, p. 2). Sudnow's experience of the modern medical management of death and dying exposed the routinization of dying and death, wherein the value of organizational efficiency was held as far more important than that of human dignity. He explained how social class affected the choice and execution of real procedures relevant to healthcare and dying in a charity hospital. He introduced the concept of social death that referred to his observation of family and staff often treating many comatose patients, technically alive, as if they were dead (Doka, 2007, p. 20). Sudnow also exposed the social inequality in the process of dying. Sudnow's work revealed that healthcare staff opted to administer their caregiving based on the patient's perceived social value: patients with low perceived social worth were much less likely to be resuscitated aggressively than patients with a high social value.

The stage theory presented in the writing of Elisabeth Kubler-Ross (*On Death and Dying*, 1969) was also developed within the sphere of the medical model hospital setting, and likewise highlighted the lonely, dehumanized isolation of dying patients. In it, Kubler-Ross proposed that dying people progressed through identifiable stages (denial, anger, bargaining, depression, acceptance) as they approached death and that each of the stages was characterized by observable behaviors and emotions. The final stage of dying, acceptance, was characterized by the dying person's acceptance of the end of life and became the goal of those who were providing their care; the concept of acceptance, along with awareness, of dying later became part of the characterization of a good death (Zimmermann, 2012). In spite of notably weak methodological foundations, Kubler-Ross's work was well-received by the general public as a welcome sort of field map for grieving caregivers and survivors who saw it as a guide to making sense of the process of dying of their loved ones.

Within this scenario, the modern hospice movement was founded in 1967 at St. Christopher's Hospice in Sydenham, outside of London, where Dr. Cicely Saunders developed her approach to managing pain and all other needs of dying patients and their families. The inpatient model hospice focused largely on those patients with advanced cancers. Because the identified trajectory of a disease like cancer makes it easier to predict death within weeks or months, pain may be managed with the use of opioids that allows the patient the possibility of living out the end of life without suffering. The hospice was staffed by an interdisciplinary team of medical, spiritual, social work, and psychological professionals.

1.3 THE ADVENT OF MODERN DEATH AWARENESS

> Dying is not only a biological affair, but a human one. The [death] movement has underscored the importance of healing the humanity wounded by illness and oncoming death. . . . Technology and competence have to be infused with compassion and benevolence and that life is not just a matter of length but of depth and quality as well.
>
> (Feifel, 1990, p. 540)

The American psychologist, Herman Feifel, broke the taboo on the subjects of death and dying, making them legitimate subjects for scientific, scholarly study. Feifel organized and chaired the first symposium on the subject, The Concept of Death and Its Relation to Behavior, in 1956 at the annual meeting of the American Psychological Association. That year, he became the first individual to be awarded a research grant from the National Institutes of Mental Health (NIMH), to study death attitudes. Feifel became known as the founder of the death psychology movement, publishing *Meanings of Death* in 1959, which became a classic in the field. He asserted that developments of an impersonal technology alienated society from traditional institutional and community supports, such that grief and dying traditions have been de-ritualized (Feifel, 1977a, p. 5). The philosophic and religious facets of Ariès's Tamed Death no longer exist to help modern society transcend death. The topic of death has, then, become uncomfortable to our culture for this and many other reasons: because we worship youth, productivity, and achievement; because death and dying have become unfamiliar to us and instead have come under the purview of the medical professionals, whose "mastery is technical" rather than human (Feifel, 1977b, p. 7). Prolongation of dying gives rise to a loss of dignity and self-esteem, as well as pain, depression, and dehumanization. Feifel pointed out that dying is not simply a biological process but a psychosocial one as well. We have altered the way in which we die: where previously persons died after acute or infectious diseases caused a more rapid death, today medical technology has prolonged death, giving rise to chronic and degenerative diseases, in hospital, nursing or convalescent homes, rather than in one's home (Feifel, 1977b).

Whereas our society witnesses disaster and death aplenty in television and movies, many are loathe to discuss death and dying. "Death is a slap in the face of the American Dream. Death refuses to die" (Morgan, 1995, p. 40). Feifel (1977b) proposed that American society, from its beginning, emphasized freedom, achievement, and a limitless future until the prospect of no future at all was brought to the fore by the World War II–ending A-bomb in Japan in 1945 (1990, p. 538), that put at risk the individuality of death, threatening a single epitaph for all of humanity. The American vision of right to life, liberty and the pursuit of happiness was dashed when the bomb was dropped. Early in the history of the United States, the national identity became one with the heroism of striving to overcome adversity in any form: of the continent's wilderness, of outer space, and of celebrity sports and media heroes. As a result, the subject of death and dying fomented hostility and the negative attitude Feifel believed was lying behind old age, the herald of death (Feifel, 1977a, p. 5). Quality of life changes for everyone with the advancement of years. The appellation of "old" has come to imply a negative value judgment (Kastenbaum, 1977, p. 40) in today's society. Our elders are often prohibited by such attitudes from discussing their feelings about death and dying and so are forced to keep these thoughts to themselves as they witness their social world, bodily image, and cognitive capacity shrink.

1.4 INSTITUTIONALIZATION, MEDICALIZATION, BUREAUCRATIZATION, PROFESSIONALIZATION

> Medicalization describes a process through which largely social issues may be redefined as medical problems, thus increasing the jurisdiction of medicine. . . . Medicalization, through disease typifications, medical authority, and the labeling of illness (or behaviors) as deviant from everyday life, has important political consequences.
>
> (Beard & Estes, 2002)

Ernest Becker's Pulitzer Prize–winning book, *The Denial of Death* (1973), has as its basic premise the idea that human civilization is an elaborate protective defense mechanism against the knowledge of mortality. This survival mechanism may be transcended through the concept of heroism, of creating something or becoming part of something eternal. A common ideology and morality arose from these values, and a battle against death became the ultimate morality play, whose starring role was technology, with a plot reinforced by the idea that the more technology, the better the healthcare. Instead, medical technology made possible the prolongation of life for those

with chronic diseases that once would have led to early death. Such prolongation of life with chronic disease has meant struggling through periods
of near death, including time in hospital in treatment for complications of
illness. The prolonged dying of individuals with low social value took place
in custodial institutions and nursing homes, removed from the view of other
members of society (Quint Benoliel & Degner, 1995).

Cutting-edge medical technology exploded in the second decade of the
21st century in most of the developed world and has succeeded in keeping
patients alive much longer than before. The research push inherent in such
a course of action treated "death as a contingent, accidental event that can
be done away with, one disease at a time" by employing the resources of
"research-ambitious medicine" (Callahan, 2005, p. S6).

End-of-life care, "or medicine practiced in order to diminish the suffering
and improve the quality of remaining life of terminally ill patients" has had
a growing role in medical care (Parker et al., 2012, p. 438). Hospitals managed the care of terminally ill patients by employing the full resources of the
ICU to effect a cure with any and all life-sustaining measures, prolonging
lives regardless of cost (Risse & Balboni, 2013). This explosion of technology evolved into the shunting of convalescing and dying patients from
hospitals to nursing homes or hospices, and now to specialized long-term
acute care hospitals. With the growing medicalization of hospitals, care of
the dying largely was abandoned to further the bottom line and hospitals
became institutions of biomedical education and research in place of care
of the dying.

The last century has witnessed unrest regarding "the sequestration and
medicalization" (Watts, 2012, p. 21) of death and dying, along with the
seeming end to the natural dignified death. Today, instead of the fear of
not existing, individuals fear being totally dependent on others, exhausting
family emotional and financial resources, and being without control and
dignity in an institution (Kearl, 1996, p. 342). In academic literature, this
disquiet was reflected in Ariès's (1974) wild savage death and in Illich's
(1976) strong critique of modern medicine, about which Illich observed
that medicine had turned death from a religious/cultural phenomenon to
a money-making one. Glaser and Strauss's (1965, 1968) seminal grounded
theory of awareness contexts, coupled with Sudnow's (1967) findings on
the social organization of dying and death in hospitals, offered powerful insights into the bureaucratic organization of death work in hospital
environments. In modern hospitals, Sudnow witnessed the routinization of
death and dying that was characterized by stringent bureaucracy in order
to minimize the disruptive possibilities of human mortality (Blauner, 1966,
referenced in Hart et al., 1998, p. 21). Dying and death were thereby shaped
through medicalization, institutionalization, and suppression that rendered
meaningless the lives of dying people in hospital. Commenting on Sudnow's
(1967) findings, Hart et al. (1998) noted that "the value of organizational
efficiency held far higher than that of human dignity" (p. 21). McNamara

and Rosenwax, in their 2007 study, found that dying for large numbers of Australians was "painful, undignified and medicalised" (p. 375). The neglect suffered by the dying and their families became the expected norm as they were left to manage by themselves.

Ivan Illich was an Austrian philosopher, Roman Catholic priest, and a critic of Western social institutions. In his book, *Limits to Medicine: Medical Nemesis, the Expropriation of Death* (1976), Illich detailed his views of modern medicine, principally that

> medical professional practice has become a major threat to health. . . .
> The so-called health-professions have an indirect sickening power—a structurally health-denying effect . . . which I designate as medical Nemesis. By transforming pain, illness, and death from a personal challenge into a technical problem, medical practice expropriates the potential of people to deal with their human condition in an autonomous way and becomes the source of a new kind of un-health."
>
> (Illich, 1976, p. 919)

Illich criticized medicine's loss of the capacity to accept suffering and death as meaningful aspects of life, eliciting a feeling of being in a state of total war against death at every stage of the life cycle. Comparable to Feifel's views of "deritualization" of death, Illich saw the devaluing of the traditional rituals surrounding death and dying as a crippling of personal and family care (Clark, 2002).

Illich viewed clinical care to be the result of intense capitalist commodity production wherein the patient as individual becomes a technological product. He proposed that the medicalization of death and dying led to new levels of social control in which a rejection of patienthood by the dying and bereaved is seen as a form of deviance (Clark, 2002). He criticized the institutionalization of dying and death that allowed physicians to attain great power and increasing influence over the lives of dying patients (Hart et al., 1998). Illich contended that the general improvement in the health of a population had no real relationship to the amount of healthcare available, but rather on such things as better awareness of sanitation on the part of the populace, coupled with improved environmental and nutritional factors. He disapproved of medicine for its prolific bureaucratization that was based on the denial of a person's need to deal with pain, sickness, and death (Bunker, 2003). By way of solutions to these problems, Illich urged individuals to return to personal responsibility for their healthcare and to turn over medical technology to laymen, to use drugs and procedures responsibly (Killeen, 1976).

Modern society has delegated almost all of its obligations to dying people exclusively to the clinical professions (Byock, 2002). While such is done with the best of intentions, this professionalization has served as a way for society to "manifest its cultural avoidance of death" (p. 284). A result of this consignment of official responsibility to doctors and nurses for society's most ill, elderly and dying, is to distance the living from difficult reminders of the looming inevitability of illness, infirmity, physical dependence, and death. People have placed all their faith in medicine's ability to cure us of anything, even of old age and dying. Medicalization of the care of the dying in postmodern medicine is symbolized by the white coats and rubber gloves of clinicians, which thereby objectifies any individual suffering an advanced or incurable illness (Byock, 2002).

In *No Place for Dying*, Chapple (2010) introduced the concept of rescue as it pertains to dying patients in hospitals. As hospital patients sought more time alive, physicians met this quest with cutting-edge use of the latest technology and thereby also met the hospitals' needs to keep their beds full: empty beds, empty pocketbooks. Clinicians went to work rescuing their patients from death, but once they were unable to accomplish a rescue and a fee, the patients had to be moved elsewhere so that the empty beds could once again become occupied and profitable. Seriously ill hospital patients who fail to get well were deemed to be officially dying and "are demoted from a first-class, rescuable status to a second-class, unrescuable status" (p. 9). Physicians must negotiate the spectrum of efforts between a patient with a future and a patient without one. "When efforts to forestall the dying process fail, professionals usually lose interest and transfer their motivation and resources elsewhere. After all, the saving of life is the paramount goal of the health professional" (Feifel, 1977b, p. 7).

The process of dying suffered by a large number of people today is painful, undignified, neglectful, and medicalized. Kaufman discussed the cultural conversation on the way death tends to occur in a community hospital as emphasizing

> discrete entities in opposition—palliation versus treatment, technology versus care, control versus powerlessness, choice versus inevitability—and ignores the lived experiences of patients, families and professionals. The actual practice of dying is revealed to be more muddled and the abstract concept of death with dignity disappears in face of the reality of hospital regulations and use of technology.
>
> (Kaufman, 1998, p. 716)

At the end of the 20th century, the location of death evolved from the home to the hospital and the responsibility for the dying individual shifted from the families and communities to the physicians and hospitals. Paramount was the full commitment to pharmaceutical, surgical, and technological interventions to prolong frail lives. Medicine became a powerful force and was most evident in the ICU in which physicians became gatekeepers of the dying process. Medicine became the primary means of confronting the problem of old age and defining it. When an elderly person becomes ill, the immediate outreach is to the tools of medicine, the institution of the hospital that is able to bring back the person from the brink of dying to a critical condition (Kaufman, 1998). The technological imperative in medicine—"to order ever more diagnostic tests, to perform procedures . . . to intervene with medication, ventilators and surgery in order to prolong life—is the most important variable in contemporary medical practice" (p. 721), even though death without the intervention of technology is valued by many. However, faced with the myriad of choices presented by biomedicine to family members of the dying, these family members do not know what to want, other than the recovery of their loved one. Such choices are created for them; they do not arise from patients' worlds of experience. "This incommensurability between medical and lay worlds of understanding is an additional source of the problem of 'death in America'" (Kaufman, 1998, p. 722; McNamara & Rosenwax, 2007). Hence, in this view, conceptions of a good death in hospital are abstract and theoretical.

As the population ages and increasingly becomes prey to severe acute illnesses and as physicians become more skilled at keeping patients alive in the ICU, the result is an increase in the number of patients highly dependent upon the delivery of the constant care needed to stay alive. These people cannot go home, to a rehabilitation facility, or to a nursing home, so many are sent to long-term acute care hospitals (LTACs), to survive, if not to recover. Patients are sent to LTACs when ICUs can do no more for them and they are faced with the continual interventions necessary to support life, while the family is confronted with the question of when to withdraw treatment. Such patients comprise a minority of ICU patients, but account for disproportionate resource use and have poor long-term outcomes (Kahn et al., 2013, p. 4). The cost of long-term acute care is substantial, about $26 billion a year in the United States, and by one estimate the number of patients in these facilities has more than tripled in the past decade to 380,000 (Kolata, 2014). Such facilities occupy a unique niche in the healthcare system.

CITATIONS: CHAPTER 1

Ariès, P. (1974). *Western attitudes towards death: From the Middle Ages to the present*. Baltimore, MD, & London: Johns Hopkins University Press.

Ariès, P. (1981). *The hour of our death*. (Helen Weaver, Ed.) (second Vintage ed.). New York: Alfred A. Knopf, Inc./Vintage Books.

Beard, R.L., & Estes, C.L. (2002). Medicalization of aging. In *Macmillan encyclopedia of aging* (pp. 883–886). New York: Macmillan Publishers. Retrieved from http://medicine.jrank.org/pages/1106/Medicalization of Aging.html.

Becker, E. (1973). *The denial of death*. New York: The Free Press/A Division of Macmillan Publishing.

Boyd, K. (1977). Attitudes to death: Some historical notes. *Journal of Medical Ethics*, 3(3), 124–128. Retrieved from www.pubmedcentral.nih.gov/articlerender.fcgi?artid=1154578&tool=pmcentrez&rendertype=abstract.

Bunker, J.P. (2003). Ivan Illich and medical nemesis. *Journal of Epidemiology & Community Health*, 57, 927. http://doi.org/10.1016/j.nedt.2011.08.003.

Byock, I. (2002). The meaning and value of death. *Journal of Palliative Medicine, 5*(2), 279–289.

Callahan, D. (2005). Death: The *"distinguished thing"*. *Improving end of life care: Why has it been so difficult?* Special Report 35, no. 6, S5–S8. Retrieved from www.ncbi.nlm.nih.gov/pubmed/16468248.

Chapple, H.S. (2010). *No place for dying*. Walnut Creek, CA: Left Coast Press.

Clark, D., & Hart, D. (2002). Between hope and acceptance: The medicalisation of dying. *BMJ, 324*(7342), 905–907.

Corr, C.A., Doka, K.J., and Kastenbaum, R. (1999). Dying and its interpreters: A review of selected literature and some comments on the state of the field. *OMEGA—Journal of Death and Dying, 39*(4), 239–259. http://doi.org/10.2190/3KGF-52BV-QTNT-UBMX.

Doka, K. (2007). Historical & contemporary perspectives on dying. In D.E. Balk (Ed.) *Handbook of thanatology* (pp. 19–25). New York & London: Routledge: Taylor & Francis Group.

Feifel, H. (1977a). Death and dying in modern America. *Death Education, 1*(1), 5–14. Retrieved from www.ncbi.nlm.nih.gov/pubmed/10306651.

Feifel, H. (1977b). Death in contemporary America. In H. Feifel (Ed.). *New meanings of death* (pp. 3–12). New York: McGraw Hill & Co.

Feifel, H. (1990). Psychology and death. Meaningful rediscovery. *The American Psychologist, 45*(4), 537–543. Retrieved from www.ncbi.nlm.nih.gov/pubmed/2186680.

Gawande, A. (2014). *Being mortal: Medicine and what matters in the end*. New York: Henry Holt & Co.

Glaser, B.G., & Strauss, A.S. (1965). *Awareness of dying*. Chicago: Aldine Publishing Co.

Glaser, B.G., & Strauss, A.S. (1968). *Time for dying*. Chicago: Aldine Publishing Co.

Gorer, G. (1955). Pornography of Death. *Encounter*, 49–52.

Hart, B., Sainsbury, P., & Short, S. (1998). Whose dying? A sociological critique of the "good death." *Mortality, 3*(1), 65–77. http://doi.org/10.1080/713685884.

Illich, I. (1976). *Limits to medicine: Medical nemesis, the expropriation of death* (2010 ed.). London & New York: Marion Boyers Publishers, Ltd.

Illich, I. (2003). Medical nemesis. *Journal of Epidemiology & Community Health, 57*(12), 919–922. http://doi.org/10.1136/jech.57.12.919.

Kahn, J.M., Werner, R.M., David, G., Ten Have, T.R., Benson, N.M., & Asch, D.A. (2013). Effectiveness of long-term acute care hospitalization in elderly patients with chronic critical illness. *Medical Care, 51*(1), 4–10. http://doi.org/10.1097/MLR.0b013e31826528a7.

Kastenbaum, R. (1977). Death and development through the lifespan. In H. Feifel (Ed.), *New meanings of death* (pp. 17–45). New York: McGraw Hill & Co.

Kaufman, S.R. (1998). Intensive care, old age, and the problem of death in America. *The Gerontologist, 38*(6), 715–725. Retrieved from www.ncbi.nlm.nih.gov/pubmed/9868851.

Kaufman, S.R., & Morgan, L.M. (2005). The anthropology of the beginnings and ends of life. *Annual Review of Anthropology, 34*(1), 317–341. http://doi.org/10.1146/annurev.anthro.34.081804.120452.

Kearl, M.C. (1996). Dying well: The unspoken dimension of aging well. *American Behavioral Scientist, 39*(3), 336–360. http://doi.org/10.1177/0002764296039003009.

Kellehear, A. (2007). *A social history of dying*. New York: Cambridge University Press.

Killeen, R.N.F. (1976). A review of Illich's Medical Nemesis. *Western Journal of Medicine, 125*(1), 67–69.

Kolata, G. (2014, June 23). Life goes on at long term care acute care hospitals. *New York Times*. Retrieved from www.nytimes.com/2014/06/24/health/life-goes-on-at-long-term-acute-care-hospitals.html?emc=eta1&_r=0.

McNamara, B., & Rosenwax, L. (2007). Mismanagement of dying. *Health Sociology Review, 16*(5), 373–383.

Morgan, J.D. (1995). Living our dying and our grieving: Historical and cultural attitudes. In H. Wass & R.A. Neimeyer (Eds.), *Dying: Facing the facts* (third ed.) (pp. 25–46). Washington, DC: Taylor & Francis.

Parker, G.D., Smith, T., Corzine, M., Mitchell, G., Schrader, S., Hayslip, B., & Fanning, L. (2012). Assessing attitudinal barriers toward end-of-life care. *The American Journal of Hospice & Palliative Care, 29*(6), 438–442. http://doi.org/10.1177/1049909111429558.

Quint Benoliel, J., & Degner, L.F. (1995). Institutional dying. In H. Wass & R.A. Neimeyer (Eds.), *Dying: Facing the facts* (third ed.) (pp. 117–142). Washington, DC: Taylor & Francis.

Risse, G.B., & Balboni, M.J. (2013). Shifting hospital-hospice boundaries: Historical perspectives on the institutional care of the dying. *The American Journal of Hospice & Palliative Care, 30*(4), 325–330. http://doi.org/10.1177/1049909112452336.

Sudnow, D. (1967). *Passing on: The social organization of dying.* Englewood Cliffs: Prentice-Hall, Inc.

Watts, T. (2012). End-of-life care pathways as tools to promote and support a good death: A critical commentary. *European Journal of Cancer Care, 21*(1), 20–30. http://doi.org/10.1111/j.1365-2354.2011.01301.x.

Zimmermann, C. (2012). Acceptance of dying: A discourse analysis of palliative care literature. *Social Science & Medicine, 75*(1), 217–224.

2 Twenty-First-Century Death
Social and Political Priorities and the Good Death

The growing proportion of elderly people in the developed world will have consequences for the economies and health care systems of these countries.

(Ellershaw et al., 2010, p. 656)

An ideal valued by many people is that of living a healthy life, followed by deterioration and death in very old age, whereas the truth is that the majority of people today die after a long period of chronic illness. The achievement of "a good death for all" is a prominent social and political priority across the Western world (Ellershaw et al., 2010). This is reflected in the reports and strategies of Western governments about enhancing end-of-life care. Consumer concerns over inadequate end-of-life care have been identified in various international health service reform agendas.

2.1 END-OF-LIFE OR "BRINK-OF-DEATH" CARE: A GOOD DEATH?

Hospice was designed to give end-of-life care, but it's turning out to be brink-of-death care.

(Byock, 2014, in Wickham, 2014)

Reforms to benefit those at the end of life ought to encompass all people sick enough to die soon, such as in answer to the no surprise question of their doctor: would you be surprised if this individual died within a year (Lynn, 2004, p. 44)? Policy makers in the developed world must achieve continuity and comprehensive care for the increasing numbers of seriously ill patients with multiple chronic conditions (Dy & Lynn, 2007; Byock, 2012; Gawande, 2014).

In the 1900s, most people died from infections and accidents in a matter of hours or days. Today, most individuals can expect to spend a few years living with substantial serious disability at the end of life. Most individuals die due to failure of a major organ (heart, lungs, kidneys, or liver), dementia, stroke, or the general frailty of old age (Lunney et al., 2004, p. 2388).

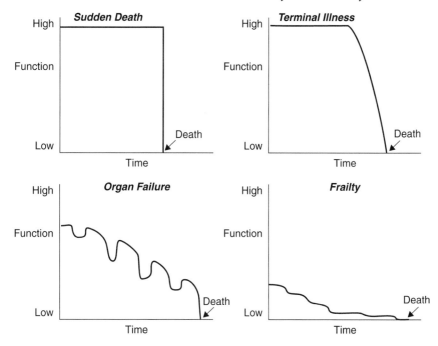

Figure 2.1   Proposed Trajectories of Dying (Lunney et al., 2002, p. 1109)

Source: Reprinted with permission by the RAND Corporation, Santa Monica, CA, the original source and copyright holder thereof: *Redefining and Reforming Health Care for the Last Years of Life* by Joanne Lynn and David M. Adamson (2003). For the full report: www.rand.org/pubs/research_briefs/RB9178.html.

Healthcare systems are not, unfortunately, designed with the view of end of life as a distinct phase of one's life rather than as a mere aberration of ill health or disability. The common pattern of care needs over time while living with fatal illnesses have been identified and may be planned for. (See Figure 2.1.) These trajectories provide a way to "describe generalities about large and discernible groups of people, each with different time courses of illness, service needs, priorities for care, and current barriers to reliably high quality care" (Dy & Lynn, 2007, p. 511; Lynn, 2004; Gawande, 2014). The first trajectory involves the maintenance of good function followed by a short period of relatively predictable decline in the last weeks or months of life, typical of cancer; the second trajectory largely represents chronic organ system failure, represented by slow decline and punctuated by dramatic exacerbations that often end in sudden death, typical of organ system failure; the third trajectory is poor long-term functional status with slow decline to death, typical of frailty and dementia (Dy & Lynn, 2007, pp. 511–12; Lynn, 2004).

When a frail, ill person at the end of life becomes critically ill, families, healthcare workers and hospital policies can easily ensure that the patient be brought back from the brink of death to critical illness. Postponing death with ventilators, medication, and surgery in order to preserve life has become the technological imperative that rules medical practice. The choices offered to patients and families reflect this technological imperative. However, just as healthcare professionals often cannot identify when the process of dying begins, patients and families do not know what treatment to continue or which to remove (Kaufman, 1998, 1999). Patients are "consumed by an all-pervasive illness, discreet disease treatment and the management of bodily life extension" (Kaufman,1999, p. 80).

2.2 WHAT POLICY HAS BEEN ACCOMPLISHED TOWARDS ACHIEVING A GOOD DEATH?

> But what is the state of dying in Britain today? Sadly, nobody can answer that question with confidence. We have reliable and detailed statistics on life expectancy, age at death, and place and cause of death, but we know little about the experience of death. For the minority who die under the care of palliative care teams it is probably good, but there is a suspicion that for the majority, who die in acute hospitals and nursing homes, the experience is bad.
>
> (Smith, 2000, p. 129)

Policy makers in developed countries are interested in knowing how and where people die as a means of meeting consumer choice in relation to such factors as dying with dignity as well as reducing costs by avoiding unnecessary and clinically futile interventions. Most deaths in developed countries now occur in the acute care setting, and these numbers are expected to increase as the population ages and more people die of chronic and complex conditions. Most of the acute care deaths will be managed by health professionals for whom end-of-life care is not the primary area of expertise and who often have no formal training in diagnosing dying.

In the acute care environment, the focus has traditionally been on "curing and prolonging life", so that tensions and challenges arose in moving care toward the palliative model of symptom management. Doing so made it difficult to support patients and families to make this transition and may explain late recognition of dying and a delay in initiating end-of-life care in hospitals. The result is suboptimal psychosocial and spiritual care, as well as poor symptom management for dying patients and their families (Phillips et al., 2011).

2.3 FACTS/FIGURES/FIXES

> If the medical profession can't serve people well throughout the entire continuum of life, we're failing. And at the moment, our health care system is failing our patients and their families, at the

end. As citizens, and as consumers of health care, we've got to insist that standards become not just better, but dramatically better.

(Byock, 2012)

In today's healthcare system in the United States, the most widely used healthcare services occur during the last phase of life, an average of two years (Lynn, 2004). Elderly Americans today are healthier than ever before, but spend their last years with serious disabilities and fatal chronic diseases that become more frequent with advancing age. "Cognitive disability and frailty are rapidly becoming dominant elements of dying in old age" (p. 9). As frail elders become more debilitated by loss of hearing, cognition, and mobility, they often become more isolated and unhappy. Chronic diseases, such as cancer, multiple organ failure, dementia, and stroke, regularly cause death in old age. In industrialized nations, the elderly exchange more time alive for such a scenario.

In the United States, the Medicare program provides health insurance for qualified elderly individuals and Medicaid covers the poor. Hospice benefits are the same for both Medicare and Medicaid. In order to access to this benefit, an individual must have a prognosis of terminal illness with a life expectancy of six months or less if the illness runs its normal course. Initially, two physicians must certify the patient as terminally ill, and no strict limit is placed on the duration of hospice care, but hospices are required to certify/recertify this prognosis. Terminally ill individuals are required to exchange their regular Medicare coverage involved with the terminal condition for the hospice benefits, so they are not then eligible to receive curative treatment.

Hospice care in the United States is predominantly provided at the routine home care level. Hospices provide interdisciplinary care and support to dying patients and their families by focusing on their physical, emotional, social, and spiritual needs. When certified, individuals are entitled to a package of services that include: physician services and nursing care; homemaker/home health aide services; social work services; counseling services (chaplain, bereavement, dietary); physical, speech, and occupational therapies; durable medical equipment; medications related to the terminal condition; medical supplies; short-term inpatient care (directly or through contract) and inpatient respite care; 24-hour availability of medical services; grief support to help the patient and family, which includes bereavement follow-up for 12 months; and any covered medically necessary and reasonable services as identified by the interdisciplinary team (Connor, 2009, p. 106).

Since its passage in 1982, the Medicare hospice benefit (MHB) has greatly improved the dying experienced of beneficiaries. Initially, the MHB provided an important means of transitioning to end-of-life care and a significant alternative to traditional care at the end of life. However, targeted reforms are needed that would allow citizens to attain the good death they want: the definition of hospice eligibility relative to the six-month prognosis mark was clinically arbitrary and practicably difficult, especially for people with non-cancer diagnoses as originally planned. Today, beneficiaries are admitted to hospice care with the full range of terminal illness whose prognoses vary widely in time span, as opposed to the more stage-oriented cancer trajectory. Limiting hospice care to patients who agree to give up disease-modifying therapy likewise enforces an artificial distinction between curative and palliative therapy and potentially impedes both enrollment and quality of care (Stephenson, 2012, p. 1684; Temel et al., 2010). A 15-site concurrent care demonstration project has been authorized by the Affordable Care Act (ACA) to allow patients to receive hospice and curative care simultaneously and is an important step towards the provision of integrating high quality palliative and end-of-life care

> into the continuum of services that beneficiaries receive. . . . This approach could ensure greater continuity of care and would be consistent with the broader aim of reorienting Medicare toward the delivery of flexible, patient centered care driven by patient's needs rather than by narrow and potentially inefficient eligibility and payment policies.
>
> (Stephenson, 2012, p. 1684, p.1685)

Older Americans 2012: Key Indicators of Well-Being (Older Americans 2012) is the sixth in a series of reports by the Federal Interagency Forum on Aging-Related Statistics (Forum) describing the overall condition of the U.S. population age 65 and over (p. iv). The report contains a special feature, "End of Life", presenting that period as a particularly difficult time for patients and their families, because many issues tend to arise, "including decisions about medical care, formal and informal caregiving, transitions in living arrangements among community, assisted living, and nursing homes, financial impacts, and whether to use advance directives and living wills" (p. 65).

The feature highlights two important aspects of end-of-life care: the place of death and the type of care received (hospice or intensive care unit/coronary care unit [ICU/CCU]) in the month prior to death. Important information is presented that sheds light on the various good death issues presented later: place of death has been indicated as a quality measure of end of life care and data indicate the increase in the rate of death at home of those 65 years old and older (Teno et al., 2013, p. 407; Paddy, 2011, p. 33). The use of hospice has increased substantially in recent years, from 19 percent of decedents in 1999 to 43 percent in 2009. The primary diagnoses associated with hospice care have changed over time, with neoplasms (cancers) accounting for 53 percent of hospice stays in 1999 and only 32 percent in 2009. The next most common primary diagnoses in 2009 were diseases of the circulatory system (19 percent) and symptoms, signs and ill-defined conditions (17 percent). Use of hospice services increased with the age of the decedent: among women, 38 percent of those dying at ages 65–74 received hospice care, compared with 49 percent of those age

85 and over. Hospice care was much more common among White decedents than among Black decedents or those of other races (Older Americans 2012).

Use of ICU/CCU services has grown more slowly, from 22 percent in 1999 to 27 percent in 2009 (Older Americans 2012, p. 66). In contrast to hospice, the use of ICU/CCU services decreased with increasing age of decedents, especially for those dying at age 85 and over. Twenty-six percent of White decedents used ICU/CCU services in the last 30 days of life compared with 32 percent of Black decedents and 33 percent of decedents of other races (pp. 65–74).

U.S. death certificates record the place of death of decedents. Where a person dies is the outcome of many factors, including cause of death, personal preferences, cultural beliefs, availability of social support, and access to medical and hospice care, among others (Older Americans 2012, p. 68; Teno et al., 2013). Most significantly, the percent of deaths that occurred while the decedent was a hospital inpatient declined over time, from 49 percent of all deaths of persons 65 and over in 1989 to 32 percent in 2009. In addition, the percent of decedents age 65 and over who died at home has increased from 15 percent in 1989 to 24 percent in 2009. The Medicare benefit, introduced in 1982, providing the incentive of lowered costs of care with the use of home hospice services, combined with the recognition that consumers prefer to die at home, has contributed to the increase in home deaths.

In the National Center for Health Statistics (NCHS) Data Brief #88, "75 Years of Mortality in the United States, 1935–2010" (Hoyert, 2012), data from the National Vital Statistics System (NVSS) from over a 75-year period included preliminary data for 2010 and examined long-term trends in mortality in the United States by age, sex, and race. Reductions in deaths and death rates are indicators of the success of public health policies and about 80 of the objectives of Healthy People 2020 concern death (U.S. Department of Health and Human Services, Healthy People 2020, www. healthypeople.gov). Although single year improvements in mortality were often small, the age-adjusted risk of dying dropped 60 percent from 1935 to 2010. Heart disease and cancer remained the first and second causes of death during that period. The decrease in death rates during those 75 years varied by age: for persons 65–74 years of age, death rates declined by 62 percent, while death rates decreased by 58 percent for those 75–84 years of age, and declined 38 percent for persons 85 years or more. The 29 percent decline in age-adjusted mortality in the earlier period from 1935 to 1954 was probably influenced by the introduction of various drugs such as antibiotics, while in the most recent period from 1969 to 2010, significant progress in the prevention, diagnosis, and treatment of cardiovascular diseases likely contributed to the 41 percent decline in age-adjusted mortality, despite cancer continuing to increase from 1969 to 1990 and chronic lower respiratory diseases continuing to increase from 1969 to 1998.

In order to help ensure that patients and families received the best possible end-of-life care, guidelines for goals of care and integrated care pathways were formulated with the aim of informing clinical decision making. Clinical care pathways, perceived as ways to standardize practice, to monitor, coordinate, and enhance care quality, to put into practice evidence-based procedures, to hold practitioners to account, and to save money, were adopted in North America and the United Kingdom in the 1990s (Watts, 2012, p. 24). End-of-life care pathways were originally promulgated to repair suboptimal care of dying people and their families. The pioneering Liverpool Care Pathway (LCP) for the Dying, led by the Marie Curie Palliative Care Institute in Liverpool, UK, is an integrated care pathway program that is targeted for improving care of the imminently dying (Bhatnagar & Joshi, 2013). The initiative has been supported and recommended as a means to translate the key principles of the hospice model of care into general healthcare settings, including hospitals, care homes, and patients' own homes. Originally the LCP, begun in the late 1990s by Ellershaw et al., was meant for the care of terminally ill cancer patients, but has since been extended to include all patients deemed to be dying. End-of-life care pathways, many of which are adaptations of the pioneering Liverpool Care Pathway (LCP) for the dying patient (Ellershaw & Ward, 2003) seek to exemplify ideal journeys through this discrete phase of palliative care into the immediate bereavement period and, as complex interventions, ensure individualized comfort care (see Figure 2.2). End-of-life care pathways have been used for a range of dying populations in a variety of acute and hospice care settings across much of the developed world. These pathways may well enhance care in the dying phase and thus facilitate a certain type of good death.

John Ellershaw of the Liverpool Care Pathway maintained that care for the dying represents a marker of Britain's commitment to providing high quality delivery of care to all (Ellershaw et al., 2010). The LCP is based on a hospice approach to death and encompasses a change in emphasis of care from life-prolonging to palliative (Hardy & Good, 2014). In 2004, the National Institute for Health and Clinical Excellence issued a list detailing the best practices in end-of-life care in the last hours and days of life:

- Current drugs are assessed and non-essential one's discontinued
- As required subcutaneous medication is prescribed according to an agreed protocol to manage pain, agitation, nausea, and vomiting and respiratory tract secretions
- Decisions are taken to discontinue inappropriate interventions
- The ability of the patient, family, and carers to communicate is assessed
- The insights of the patient, family, and carers into the patient's condition are identified
- Religious and spiritual needs of the patient, family, and carers are assessed

Principles of a good death:

- To know when death is coming, and to understand what can be expected
- To be able to retain control of what happens
- To be afforded dignity and privacy
- To have control over pain relief and other symptom control
- To have choice and control over where death occurs (at home or elsewhere)
- To have access to information and expertise of whatever kind is necessary
- To have access to any spiritual or emotional support required
- To have access to hospice care in any location, not only in hospital
- To have control over who is present and who shares the end
- To be able to issue advance directives which ensure wishes are respected
- To have time to say goodbye, and control over other aspects of timing
- To be able to leave when it is time to go, and not to have life prolonged pointlessly

Figure 2.2   Principles of a Good Death (Smith, 2000, p. 129)

- Means of informing family and carers of the patient's impending death are identified
- Family and carers are given appropriate written information
- The general practitioner is made aware of the patient's condition
- A plan of care is explained and discussed with the patient, family, and carers

(Quoted in Ellershaw et al., 2010, p. 456)

Whereas initial reception for the LCP was positive and adopted worldwide, in July 2013 the unfavorable results of an independent review into the LCP led by Baroness Julia Neuberger were published. The government accepted the review's recommendation and advised that NHS hospitals should phase out the use of the LCP over the next 6–12 months. The review concluded that "although good in principle, there was the risk that because of the focus on documentation, the LCP could be used as a tick box exercise and paradoxically lead to worse care if used incorrectly or incompetently" (Hardy & Good, 2014, p. 313). The report also found that "where the LCP was operated by well-trained, well-resourced and sensitive clinicians, many relatives felt that their loved ones had had good deaths" (Kelly, 2014, p. 37).

In Britain, the End of Life Care Strategy describes a good death as "being treated as an individual, with dignity and respect; being without pain and other symptoms; being in familiar surroundings; and being in the company of close family and/or friends" (Department of Health [DH] 2008, in Paddy, 2011, p. 33). A particular aim is to meet the care and social needs of adults at the end of life, including any preference over where they die.

The Economist Intelligence Unit (2010) published *The Quality of Death: Ranking End-of-Life Care Across the World*. Advancements in healthcare have been responsible for most quality of life gains and humans are living longer and more healthfully. However, the quality of death proves to be a much different case. Curative medicine often is at odds with the demands of end-of-life palliative care in which recovery is not likely, so that the task of minimizing suffering falls to the physician or caregiver. Few nations, including rich ones with cutting-edge healthcare systems, do not implement palliative care strategies into their overall healthcare policies, even in face of growing longevity and of aging populations, who will create a growing demand for end-of-life care. The key findings of this report, most relative to this discussion of end-of-life care as it impacts on a good death, are that the United Kingdom leads the world in most indicators of quality of death and that state funding of end-of-life care is limited and often prioritizes conventional medicine, thereby putting palliative care at a disadvantage. A possible solution to this conundrum has been offered by the United States Institute of Medicine's 2014 recommendations to the government of ways to improve the delivery of healthcare.

Policymakers in industrialized countries have a long road to travel to improve public health matters and delivery of optimal end-of-life healthcare for the terminal elderly of the 21st century: the integration of high quality palliative and end-of-life care; the assurance of better continuity of care; the delivery of patient-centered care driven by patient's needs; the expansion of medical education about dying to medical students; and the promotion of public health education to the general public about healthcare and end-of-life decision making.

CITATIONS: CHAPTER 2

Bhatnagar, S., & Joshi, S. (2013). "A good death"—Sequence (not stigma), to an enigma called life: Case report on end-of-life decision making and care. *The American Journal of Hospice & Palliative Care, 30*(7), 626–627. http://doi.org/10.1177/1049909112458962.

Byock, I. R. (2012). A better way to die. Retrieved from www.aarp.org/health/doctors-hospitals/info-03–2012/palliative-care-ira-byock-author-speaks.html.

Connor, S. R. (2009). U.S. hospice benefits. *Journal of Pain and Symptom Management, 38*(1), 105–109. http://doi.org/10.1016/j.jpainsymman.2009.04.012.

Dy, S., & Lynn, J. (2007). Getting services right for those sick enough to die. *BMJ (Clinical Research Ed.), 334*(7592), 511–513.

Economist Intelligence Unit. (2010). *The quality of death: Ranking end-of-life care across the world.* London: The Economist.

Ellershaw, J., Dewar, S., & Murphy, D. (2010). Achieving a good death for all. *BMJ (Clinical Research Ed.), 341*(7774), 656–658. Retrieved from www.ncbi.nlm.nih.gov/pubmed/20847021.

Ellershaw, J., & Ward, C. (2003). Care of the dying patient: The last hours or days of life. *BMJ, 326*(7379), 30–34.

Federal Interagency Forum on Aging-Related Statistics (2012). *Older Americans 2012: Key indicators of well-being.* Washington, DC: U.S. Government Printing Office. Retrieved from www.agingstats.gov.

Gawande, A. (2014). *Being mortal: Medicine and what matters most in the end.* New York: Henry Holt & Co.

Hardy, J.R., & Good, P. (2014). A good death in hospital. *Internal Medicine Journal, 44*(4), 313–314. http://doi.org/10.1111/imj.12378.

Hoyert, D.L. (2012). 75 years of mortality in the United States, 1935–2010. *NCHS Data Brief,* no. 88, 1–8. Retrieved from www.ncbi.nlm.nih.gov/pubmed/22617094.

Kaufman, S.R. (1998). Intensive care, old age, and the problem of death in America. *The Gerontologist, 38*(6), 715–725. Retrieved from www.ncbi.nlm.nih.gov/pubmed/9868851.

Kaufman, S.R. (1999). The clash of meanings: Medical narrative and biographical story at life's end. *Generations, 23*(4), 77–82.

Kelly, C.M.J. (2014). What is a Good Death? *The New Bioethics, 20*(1), 35–52. http://doi.org/10.1179/2050287714Z.00000000042.

Lunney, J.R., Lynn, J., Foley, D.J., Lipson, S., & Guralnik, J.M. (2004). Patterns of functional decline at the end of life. *JAMA, 289*(18), 2387–2392.

Lynn, J. (2004). *Sick to death and not going to take it anymore! Reforming health care for the last years of life.* Berkeley & Los Angeles, CA: University of California Press.

Paddy, M. (2011). Influence of location on a good death. *Nursing Standard, 26*(1), 33–36. http://doi.org/10.7748/ns2011.09.26.1.33.c8693.

Phillips, J.L., Halcomb, E.J., & Davidson, P.M. (2011). End-of-life care pathways in acute and hospice care: An integrative review. *Journal of Pain and Symptom Management, 41*(5), 940–955. http://doi.org/10.1016/j.jpainsymman.2010.07.020.

Smith, R. (2000). A good death: An important aim for health services and for us all. *BMJ, 320*(7228), 129–130.

Stephenson, D. (2012). Growing pains for the Medicare Hospice Benefit. *The New England Journal of Medicine, 367*(18), 1683–1685. http://doi.org/10.1056/NEJMp1209693.

Temel, J.S., Greer, J.A., Muzikansky, A., Gallagher, E.R., Admane, S., Jackson, V.A., . . . Lynch, T.J. (2010). Early palliative care for patients with metastatic non-small-cell lung cancer. *The New England Journal of Medicine, 363*(8), 733–742. http://doi.org/10.1056/NEJMoa1000678.

Teno, J.M., Gozalo, P.L., Bynum, J.P.W., Leland, N.E., Miller, S.C., Morden, N.E., . . . Goodman, D.C. (2013). Change in end-of-life care for Medicare beneficiaries. *JAMA, 309*(5), 470–477.

Watts, T. (2012). End-of-life care pathways as tools to promote and support a good death: A critical commentary. *European Journal of Cancer Care, 21*(1), 20–30. http://doi.org/10.1111/j.1365-2354.2011.01301.x.

Wickham, S.K. (2014, January 11). Hospice care: Limited end-of-life care fails to take into account such care may prolong life. *New Hampshire Sunday News.* Retrieved from www.unionleader.com/apps/pbcs.dll/article?AID=/20140112/NEWS12/140119839/0/sports07#sthash.TD5wfrlw.dpuf.

3 End-of-Life Care and the Good Death

> The barest essential components of human care at the end of life would seem to be the following: The provision of shelter. . . . The provision of hygiene. . . . Assistance with elimination. . . . The offering of food and drink and assistance with eating. . . . The keeping of company, nonabandonment . . . symptom management, the alleviation of suffering.
>
> (Byock, 2002, p. 284)

End-of-life care is medicine practiced in order to "diminish the suffering and improve the quality of the remaining life of terminally ill patients" (Parker et al., 2012) and has had a growing role over the past few decades in helping to ensure a good death. This type of medical care is different than that given at other times of life and ought to be recognized prospectively. The aim is to provide care that is supportive and focused on control of symptoms, particularly pain, as opposed to being invasive and aimed at extending life (Lamont, 2005; Steinhauser, Christakis, et al., 2000). A conceptual model of quality end-of-life care could be achieved when healthcare professionals "(1) ensure desired physical comfort and emotional support, (2) promote shared decision making, (3) treat the dying person with respect, (4) provide information and emotional support to family members, and (5) coordinate care across settings" (Teno et al., 2001, p. 88). Patients at the end of life face threats not only to physical well-being, but also to emotional and spiritual integrity.

3.1 CANCER AND END-OF-LIFE (EOL) CARE

> Over the centuries, cancer has had a particular horror attached to it because it was seen as certain death and it carried the fear and mystique of a disease whose cause and cure were unknown.
>
> (Holland, 2001, p. 458)

In many ways, globally, the story of modern end-of-life care is the story of cancer. Many people believe that cancer is the prototype of fatal illness.

While cancer is the second largest cause of death in the United States, behind heart failure, the trajectory of this disease follows a more predictable course that allows easier identification of patients near the end of life. Cancer is not merely a single disease, but over 150 distinct ones that are classified into four major groupings: carcinomas, sarcomas, leukemias and lymphomas (Tucci, 2010).

The fear of cancer can be traced far back to medieval times when advanced disease was first diagnosed and rapidly followed by death. By the 1990s, a cancer diagnosis was treatable by chemotherapy and radiotherapy and survival time was lengthened, but the fear of the disease and the expectation of its attendant pain and suffering grew. Researchers have found that the degree of distress patients experienced was related more to the threat to life of cancer than to the objective prognosis (Lee & Loiselle, 2012).

Until the second quarter of the 20th century, a diagnosis of cancer was viewed as equivalent to a death sentence. To reveal a diagnosis was considered cruel and inhumane, motivating the patient to lose hope. Cancer was considered a stigma that extended to the family and was spoken about in whispers (Holland, 2004; Jacobson et al., 2012) until the 1940s when the American Cancer Society initiated a partnership between medicine and government and the National Cancer Institute was founded. Cancer, its prevention and treatment, became a major health priority and has remained so until the present. In 1970, Nixon declared war on cancer and the National Institute of Health took up the cause. From then on, militaristic metaphors and the imagery of struggle entered popular usage and it has become common to "view the language of cancer in popular and scientific culture as militaristic" (Seale, 2001, p. 308). In a qualitative study, struggle talk, or "doing the good death", was often articulated as not giving up and fighting for your life (Broom & Cavanagh, 2010, p. 871). In 1978, Susan Sontag published an analysis of illness as metaphor and noted the common usage of terms like fight, battle, crusade, victims, victory, and the war against cancer (in Seale, 2001, p. 308).

Modern cancer care began with the establishment of hospice in 1967 at St. Christopher's in Sydenham. The ways in which hospice care was developed around the world was influenced by the predictable trajectory of cancer. Cancer researchers conduct hundreds of clinical trials at the major centers of excellence and present findings at national conferences and in scholarly publications (Doka, 2010, pp. 3–12). The other major chronic diseases, such as heart failure, COPD, and renal disease, are beginning to adapt many strategies from cancer research in their own research and treatment. However, most elderly Americans die by the failure of a major organ, or by dementia, stroke, or the frailty of old age, wherein the timing of death is not predictable and comes unexpectedly.

Callahan (2005) described Ariès's tame death, its beliefs that any individual death was a loss to the community itself and that "how people died and the meaning of death were inextricably blended" (p. S5). Callahan supposed that such loss of life and its attendant mourning rituals came to a halt sometime during the 1950s–60s, when lifesaving drugs and technologies gave physicians a way to approach death aggressively. He recalled that the "quality of life, the actual prognosis, or the pain induced by zealous treatment were all but irrelevant" (p. S6). A backlash in the late 1960s was marked by complaints against the useless and painful treatments, abandonment at the end of life, and death of patients swallowed up in a cocoon of tubes and monitors. Such complaints occasioned reform efforts focusing on means to improve end-of-life care, the most salient of which was the SUPPORT study.

3.2 END-OF-LIFE CARE, THE SUPPORT STUDY, AND THE GOOD DEATH

> If death is seen as a failure rather than as an important part of life then individuals are diverted from preparing for it and medicine does not give the attention it should to help dying people die a good death. We need a new approach to death.
>
> (Smith, 2000, p. 129)

The objectives of the landmark 28-million-dollar SUPPORT study (Study to Understand Prognoses and Preferences for Outcomes and Risks of Treatment, 1995) were to improve end-of-life decision making by reducing the frequency of a mechanically supported, painful, and prolonged process of dying. The SUPPORT study was conducted at five teaching hospitals in the United States with a total of 9,105 seriously ill hospitalized adults. The study partners first conducted a two-year prospective observational study (Phase I) of 4,301 severely ill patients, who were not expected to live more than six months, which confirmed substantial shortcomings in care for seriously ill hospitalized adults. The SUPPORT study concluded that the dying process in hospital was unsatisfactory: only 47 percent of physicians knew when their patients wanted to avoid CPR; 39 percent of patients spent over ten days or more before death in the ICU; 46 percent of do-not-resuscitate orders (DNRs) were written within the last two days of life even though 79 percent already had a DNR in place; and families reported that 50 percent of conscious patients experienced moderate to severe pain in the last three days of life (Schroeder, 1999).

A second two-year randomized clinical trial study (Phase II), based on the Phase I findings, failed to improve care or patient outcomes. Previous studies had likewise reported that communication between physicians and their patients was absent or occurred only during a crisis. The SUPPORT partners hypothesized that increased communication and understanding of prognoses and preferences would result in earlier treatment decisions, reductions in time spent in undesirable states before death, and reduced resource use (SUPPORT Principal Investigators, 1995, p. 1591). The Phase II intervention had supplied the

> . . . physicians reliable prognostic information and timely reports of patient and surrogate perceptions, the two most important factors cited recently by physicians when considering life-support decisions for critically ill patients. The intervention nurse also undertook time-consuming discussions, arranged meetings, provided information, supplied forms, and did anything else to encourage the patient and family to engage in an informed and collaborative decision-making process with a well-informed physician.
>
> (SUPPORT Principal Investigators, 1995, p. 1591)

Despite providing improved information, enhanced conversation and an explicit effort to encourage the use of outcome data and preferences in decision making, the results of Phase II of SUPPORT were completely ineffectual. The investigators had hoped that, "when confronted with life-threatening illness, the patient and family would be included in discussions, realistic estimates of outcome would be valued, pain would be treated, and dying would not be prolonged" (p. 1597). When the code was broken, the investigators were astonished to find that little difference existed between the experimental and the control group. Phase II of SUPPORT documented that patients still often died painful, prolonged deaths, while receiving unwanted, expensive, invasive care: quantity of life rather than quality of life, such that "patients' emotional suffering at the end of life can be profound, yet physicians are too frequently ill equipped to address this suffering" (Steinhauser, Christakis, et al., 2000, p. 2476). SUPPORT challenged the conventional wisdom that merely providing information to physicians made a difference in process or outcomes of care (Schroeder, 1999, pp. 780–1). Even though the effectiveness of the intervention was a disappointment, "the SUPPORT study provided a scientifically and medically reputable critique of how patients died in American hospitals" and served to legitimize further investments within academic medicine that began the transformation of standard practices of end-of-life care (DelVecchio Good et al., 2004, p. 941).

As the global population of baby boomers has aged, the role of end-of-life care in medicine has become more important today than ever before. However, as seen in the results of SUPPORT, patients and families prefer medical care during this particular period to be home-based and focused on improving patients' symptoms with minimally invasive means rather than with hospital-based acute care. Unfortunately, the reverse is often true. In 1997, the United States Institute of Medicine issued the report *Approaching Death*, which observed: "In the United States, death at home in the care of family has been widely superseded by an institutional, professional, and technological process of dying" (IOM, 1997, p. 33).

In summary, the SUPPORT study highlighted four major shortcomings in the care of dying or of seriously ill patients:

1. The patient and family were not included in discussions of goals of care.
2. Realistic estimates of outcomes in order to facilitate more rapid decision making were not valued.
3. Pain was not appropriately treated.
4. Dying was prolonged.

Put another way: A good death was revealed to *not* be dying a prolonged death while undergoing aggressive, unwanted treatment, frequently on life support systems, in an acute care hospital, often suffering severe pain and fatigue, shortness of breath (dyspnea), and dysphoria (Lynn et al., 1997).

3.3 END-OF-LIFE CARE AND "THE PROMISE OF A GOOD DEATH"

In 1997, the Institute of Medicine provided a definition of a good death:

> People should be able to expect and achieve a decent or good death—*one that is free from avoidable distress and suffering for patients, families, and caregivers; in general accord with patients and families wishes; and reasonably consistent with clinical, cultural, and ethical standards*
>
> (IOM, 1997, p. 5; italics in original)

All of the parameters presented in IOM's definition are reasonable; however, such definitions are vague and difficult to translate into clinical practice. In any event, such definitions do not go far enough, in an explicit way, toward defining what patients and their families are concerned with in end-of-life care (Emanuel & Emanuel, 1998, p. SII21).

The Emanuel and Emanuel (1998) article provided a schema adapted from the Commonwealth-Cummings project on the quality of care at the end of life, which most significantly characterized dying as a multidimensional experience. The schema, shown in the framework for a good death in Figure 3.1, expands the considerations of death beyond the physical and psychological symptoms a dying person experiences. This "comprehensive list of modifiable dimensions" (p. SII22) together comprises the possibilities within the complete framework inherent in creating a good death Four critical components, shown at the bottom of the framework, synthesize the dying experience:

1. The Fixed Characteristics of the patient include his or her Sociodemographic Characteristics (age, education, ethnicity, race) and Clinical Status (the disease and prognosis).

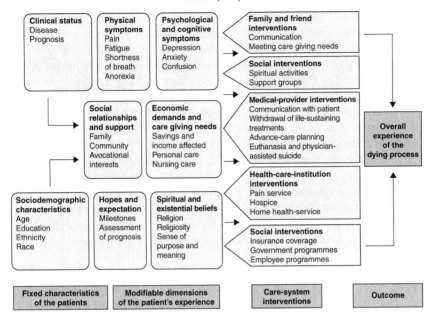

Figure 3.1   The Promise for a Good Death (Emanuel & Emanuel, 1998, p. SII22)

2. The Modifiable dimensions of the patient's experience produced by the Fixed characteristics include the qualities of Hopes and expectations that encompass patient milestones and his or her assessment of prognosis, and the element of Spiritual and existential beliefs (religion/religiosity, sense of purpose and meaning). Related to the Clinical status category is assessment of the Physical symptoms (pain, fatigue, etc.) and the Psychological and cognitive symptoms (depression, anxiety, confusion). Also represented are two effects that are associated with both the Sociodemographic characteristics and the Clinical status: the patient's Social relationships and support (family, community, etc.) and the Economic demands and caregiving needs (savings/income, personal and nursing care); Hopes and expectations (milestones and assessment of prognosis); and Spiritual and existential beliefs (religion/religiosity, sense of purpose and meaning) (Emanuel & Emanuel, 1998, p. SII22).

3. The third critical component is the resulting Care-system Interventions delineated by the five items that arise from the previous qualities: Social interventions such as insurance coverage, government programs, and employee programs; Health-care-institutions interventions including pain service, hospice, home health-service; Medical-provider interventions entailing communication with patient, withdrawal of life-sustaining treatments, advance care planning, euthanasia, and

PAS; Social interventions that include spiritual activities and support groups; and Family and friend interventions such as communication and meeting caregiving needs. These are potential interventions to be used where appropriate, but not all interventions are appropriate in all cases. The framework emphasizes that "caring for dying patients occurs within an institutional system that can significantly affect the quality of the dying experience by development of specialized care teams and facilities, institutional affiliations and reimbursement policies" (Emanuel & Emanuel, 1998, p. SII22).

4. All of the items represented on the framework, and each in their own crucial way, evolve into the fourth sought-after criterion that represents the agglomeration of the insights of end-of-life care: the Outcome, the final summation of all the modifiable criteria within the framework, which results in the Overall experience of the dying process, and which hopefully shall be considered a good death.

These four criteria contain amongst them a substantial range of specific concerns, each of which contains modifiable aspects of any patient's experience. Not only does the framework assess physical symptoms but also the other six items of the Modifiable Dimensions criteria, and may be used to define and measure suffering (p. SII23). Interventions for achieving a good death entail gaining control over pain; assessing and improving upon the effects of depression and psychological distress; improving on the economic adverse effects on caregivers; understanding the types of social supports dying patients rely on; obtaining data on spiritual and existential issues affecting dying patients; and learning the way to best handle denial of prognosis that impedes planning for death and leads to unrealistic requests for treatments.

Ultimately, a good death means different things to different people and a decision to use or not to use possible interventions: withdrawal of life-sustaining treatments; advance care planning; or hospice (Emanuel & Emanuel, 1998).

3.4 PAIN AND SUFFERING

> Suffering is experienced by persons, not merely by bodies. . . . Physicians' failure to understand the nature of suffering can result in medical intervention that (though technically adequate) not only fails to relieve suffering but becomes a source of suffering itself.
>
> (Cassel, 1982, p. 639)

Having written these words in 1982, Cassel observed that patients were well-acquainted with pain but that physicians were not: "The relief of suffering, it would appear, is considered one of the primary ends of medicine by patients and lay persons, but not by the medical profession" (p. 640). This was amply revealed by the SUPPORT study. The concern of traditional medicine was with the body, the objective physical aspects of disease (Byock, 1996), whereas patients began to demand attention to the subjective aspects of the person and mind.

Cassel (1982) made three points about suffering: first, suffering is experienced by persons, whose personhood is associated with mind, spirit, and the subjective, as well as with many other facets, the ignorance of which causes suffering: "The understanding of the place of the person in human illness requires a rejection of the historical dualism of mind and body" (p. 640). Second, suffering extends beyond the physical manifestations of acute pain and can be therefore defined as "the state of severe distress associated with events that threaten the intactness of the person" (p. 640). Cassel's third point has to do with suffering as any aspect of the person and their personhood.

The concept of suffering is usually linked with that of pain: the greater the pain, the greater the suffering. When people suffer from pain, Cassel found that clinically they do so because they feel out of control, overwhelmed by the pain, or ignorant of the source of the pain, or when the meaning of the pain is dire and when it is chronic, and hence a threat to their continued existence, to their integrity as persons. This is the relation of pain to suffering, because suffering is relieved when pain is controlled (p. 641). Likewise, the concept of suffering has a temporal element, in that its source influences the person's perception of future events: bodies do not construct meaning and do not have sense of the future, only persons do (Cassel & Rich, 2010, p. 436).

When the biotechnology imperative burgeoned and co-opted the spirit of healthcare, suffering patients and their families/caregivers reacted, fighting for, in a sense, a good death, one in which the losses of personhood they suffered might be reclaimed. Partly, they realized that although medical care can reduce the impact of sickness, inattentive care can increase the disruption caused by illness (Cassel, 1982, p. 642). Clinicians need to learn what causes patient suffering, and the only way to accomplish that is to ask the sufferer; physicians can then assist in recovery from suffering by lending strength, even if only by being present (Cassel, 1982; Byock, 1996).

3.5 COMMUNICATION OF DIAGNOSIS, PROGNOSIS, AND TREATMENT OPTIONS

> In clinical medicine, the end of life can be thought of as the period preceding an individual's natural death from a process that is unlikely to be arrested by medical care.
>
> (Lamont, 2005, 13)

Physical, psychosocial, and existential suffering can cause in terminally ill individuals the desire for hastened death (DHD), and this may even be considered, in such circumstances, a good death. Schroepfer (2007) sought to identify events common to the dying process that potentially can lead vulnerable, terminally ill individuals to experience physical and/or psychosocial suffering that makes DHD more desirable (p. 137). At issue here is not DHD in and of itself, but the four critical events of the dying process that were identified in this study that can lead such terminal elders to consider DHD: "1) perceived, insensitive communication of a terminal diagnosis; 2) experiencing unbearable physical pain; 3) unacknowledged feelings regarding undergoing chemotherapy or radiation treatment; 4) dying in a distressing environment" (pp. 139–40). Improving upon the difficulties of communicating diagnoses, prognoses, treatment options, and care placement is a crucial component of delivering quality of life in end-of-life care and moving towards assuring a good death.

The most unfulfilled promises of end-of-life care, according to patient families, has been the lack of emotional support and availability provided by physicians, their reluctance to discuss death, and the mismanagement of the patient's pain and suffering. About one of four family members "reported concerns with physician communication regarding medical decision making" (Teno et al., 2004, p. 91; Schroepfer, 2007). In the large study by Teno et al. (2004), bereaved family members voiced significant concerns regarding the end-of-life issues of their loved ones. Despite place of death in hospital or nursing homes, those whose relatives received home hospice care voiced greater satisfaction. Key findings of the study were that family members reported high rates of unmet needs for symptom management; concerns about physician communication about medical decision making; a lack of emotional support for themselves; and a belief that their dying family member was not always treated with respect (Teno et al., 2004, p. 92). The authors saw this as a public health problem that needed attention before the onslaught of the baby boom generation wreaked significant havoc with the potential provision of a good death.

Diagnosis

> . . . . What is a diagnosis? It has three parts: a name for an organic disorder, what a doctor does to explain a patient's complaints, and a method of management. . . . Diagnosis is not simply a set of terms, but a series of problem-solving assessments.
>
> (Weisman, 1974, p. 19)

Living at the end of life is a complex personal experience. The diagnosis of a life-threatening illness rocks the world of a patient and family, who then each day face the specter of impending death and an uncertain future. A study by Farber et al. (2003) undertook a qualitative analysis comparing four primary issues of quality end-of-life (EOL) care: "awareness of impending death, management/coping with daily living while attempting to maintain the management regimen, relationship fluctuations, and the personal experiences associated with facing EOL" (p. 19).

The salient finding of this study was that terminally ill people seek to live their lives as fully as possible until death overtakes them, rather than marking time and waiting to die. The reality of a diagnosis elicits, on the part of the patient and family, the need to make decisions that are congruent with their singular goals and values; healthcare professionals arrive at the diagnosis confronted by the objective of controlling the disease in order to offer hope and prolongation of life. Hence, a clash of values and purposes may be in the making for the two parties involved: quality or quantity of life? Medical perspective versus the patient's lived experiences, wants and needs (Farber et al., 2003)? The cultural perspectives of each of the stakeholders in this complex drama must become concordant in order to arrive at a good death.

When a terminal patient is in distress, a physician's immediate reaction is to see the situation through the medical lens that entails cure and prolongation of life (Proulx & Jacelon, 2004, p. 118). The diagnosis of dying is a complex set of decisions (Ellershaw & Ward, 2003), and efforts are underway to establish a set of diagnostic indicators to standardize such decisions (Kennedy et al., 2014). Analysis within a study by Kennedy et al. (2014) aimed at determining how physicians judge patients to be in the final hours of life, reinforced the theme of the difficulty of diagnosing death, thus making it ever more difficult to achieve a good death. The reverence for and availability of biotechnology, coupled with any hope of improvement, contributes to the tendency of continuing unnecessary interventions into the last days of life: "not knowing when dying begins and when death is likely to occur commonly results in the prescribing of active, life-prolonging treatments right up until death" (Proulx, 2004, p. 118). The predictability of the dying phase—the last days or hours of life—is clearest to diagnose in cancer patients (Ellershaw & Ward, 2003; Kaufman, 1999), but is not always as clear in other chronic, incurable diseases. The most important element of diagnosing dying is that the multi-professional care team be in agreement that the patient is likely to die. Acknowledging the possibility of death allows for a realistic plan of care to be discussed and the family/caregivers to express their preferences (Kennedy et al., 2014).

Prognosis, Communication, and Goals of Care

The disparity between the preferred and the actual forms of care at the end of life often have to do with the difficulty of healthcare professionals to diagnose the signs of impending death in order to make an accurate prognosis and to deliver appropriate care (Lamont, 2005). Invariably, healthcare providers overestimate survival at the end of life. Physicians formulate prognoses, the estimates of survival, about their patients with unconscious optimism and still further conscious optimism in those they communicate to their patients. In fact, a study by Lamont and Christakis (2001) compared the estimates by doctors of length of survival of almost 500 terminally ill patients and then followed the patients. The findings showed that 63 percent of doctors overestimated their patient's survival time, while just 17 percent underestimated it. Physicians' views proved to be unrealistic, such that most are reluctant to provide a specific prognosis. Improvement in both prognostic accuracy and prognostic communication "has the potential to improve the timely awareness by both physicians and patients of the onset of the end of life" (Lamont, 2005, p. S18). The result may favor a shift to home-based, symptom-guided care and away from hospital-based, life-extending care (p. S18) and, one may hope, towards a good death.

Accurate prognosis has been found to benefit patients by facilitating end-of-life planning, including discussions about life-prolonging treatment preferences and the establishment of do-not-resuscitate orders (Mack et al., 2008). The uncertainty and inaccuracy of prognoses also were found to allow for the possibility of the coping aspect of hope—for remission, cure, new treatment (Johnson, 2007). An accurate prognosis has a significant, positive impact on the quality of life of patients with advanced cancer and their caregivers. Chochinov (2000) found a significant relationship between the communication of an accurate prognosis and the reduced psychological distress in patients with advanced cancer.

How may these complex life and death decisions be achieved? Patients, families, caregivers, and healthcare professionals are tied to one another in making complex life and death decisions. Patients and families arrive bearing only their personal human experience—truly strangers in a strange land—while clinicians contribute the power of the objectivity of information and statistics, retaining the roadmap, so to speak, of the unfamiliar terrain. This dichotomy of experience and imbalance of power needs to be negotiated and resolved by good communication—speaking and listening to one another, the clinician helping to navigate the steep learning curve of the end-of-life care decisions facing the patient and family. Good communication is the heart of all medicine. Patients experience a double need: to know and understand as well as to be known and understood, while clinicians are faced with communicating empathy to patients newly diagnosed with a life-limiting illness (Van Vliet & Epstein, 2014). The parties must learn how to relate to one another in a collaborative way on the particularly troubling question of facing mortality (Best et al., 2014; Farber et al., 2003). Effective communication with healthcare providers is critical for helping family caregivers understand, manage, and derive meaning during the changes that accompany a life-limiting illness. The timely communication of information and meaningful discussion of disease progression can help families prepare for the advanced stages of an illness and an approaching death (Waldrop et al., 2012). In preparing for the end of life, good communication between patients and clinicians may help prepare patients not only practically but also personally and socially in relation to the dying process and the welfare of their families (Wentlandt et al., 2011).

Concerns about the communication skills of physicians are longstanding. Effective communication skills with patients take time and what is called "active listening" (Levinson & Pizzo, 2011, p. 1802). Delivering excellent medical care—patient-centered or relationship-centered or "biopsychosocial" care—requires both sophisticated scientific knowledge as well as sophisticated communication skills to understand the patients' needs, to address compassionately their feelings and concerns, and to educate them regarding their options of care. In the biopsychosocial approach, disease and illness are seen as mutually influencing one another, calling on "the physician in partnership with the patient to flexibly and mindfully select the dimensions of a patient's problem that are most relevant" (Frankel & Quill, 2005, p. 414). Physicians have typically applied themselves to the task of eliciting information from patients, a "physician-centered interview", rather than conducting a "patient-centered interview". Empirical evidence supports the effectiveness of patient-centered interviews that involve the doctors making eye contact with the patient, asking open-ended questions, responding to affect, and demonstrating empathy. Such communication techniques enhance disclosure of the issues of concern to a patient, decrease anxiety, assess depression, and improve a patient's well-being and the level of the patient's and the family's satisfaction with the treatment (Morrison & Meier, 2004)

The oncologist Lodovico Balducci (2012) suggested ways to implement issues of prognosis and its communication (p. iii56). He described effective open communication with the dying patient that includes a collaboration amongst healthcare personnel and the patient and the family, placing the greatest responsibility in the hands of the providers to identify and define patient wishes and cultural values. Reflective listening by the provider entails the need:

1. To notice the patient's demeanor and non-verbal communications
2. To understand the meaning of dignity to the patient that allows for that person to take ownership and control of their disease
3. To deliver the news of an imminent death at a time when the patient is ready and in a manner that is congruent with that patient's emotional and spiritual condition at that time
4. To understand that countenance and non-verbal responses are always more meaningful than the patient's own words
5. To adapt each communication to fit each patient's circumstances in life
(Balducci, 2012, p. iii56)

Prognosis is a difficult situation and its communication is an art in itself: what and how much to tell the patient and when to discuss such a sensitive topic? How much does a patient and their family caregivers want to know about the diagnosis and when should this information be delivered? Physicians have the obligation, informed consent, to communicate effectively and appropriately to the patient/family the details and extent of the diagnosis, prognosis, and range of possible treatments. Negotiating this terrain is a difficult first step in communicating with the patient and family: often, the patient/family is ambivalent about knowing the truth and the physician may be ambivalent about how and when to communicate such sensitive information. In the situation of knowledge of an incurable illness, often family/caregivers have claimed to have not been told, or have been told very late to avail themselves of the benefits of hospice care, of saying goodbyes, and of making personal and financial arrangements. Frequently, even when physicians inform the patient/family of an incurable illness, the patient/family does not agree with or accept the prognosis. Given the diversity of views and preferences for information of patients/family caregivers, a uniform method of communicating prognoses at the end of life may not be possible (Cherlin et al., 2005).

Family members/caregivers play important roles in end-of-life treatment decisions, and depend upon clinicians for an understanding of treatments and their alternatives, including use of hospice. However, communication with healthcare professionals often consists of infrequent discussion of hospice by physicians, inadequacy in physician understanding of patient preferences and shared decision making, and poor agreement on whether prognosis information was discussed among patient, family members, and physicians (Cherlin et al., 2005, p. 1177). This study showed that effective communication amongst these players is a critical element of high quality end-of-life care whose effectiveness would optimize provision of a good death.

Over 50 years ago, doctors typically did not inform patients of their diagnoses (Chochinov et al., 2000), a practice which today would clash with the ethical provisions of patient autonomy (Lamont & Christakis, 2001). Today, patients are routinely informed about their diagnoses, but physicians have issues about making and delivering prognoses, despite patient preference to the contrary. Knowing the facts of one's prognosis for survival, especially at the end of life, impacts crucially on medical and nonmedical decisions of further treatment (Butow et al., 2002). Studies have shown that discrepancies exist between doctors' prognostic estimates and the optimistic estimates of patients: in patients with terminal cancer, optimistic prognostic estimates may lead to choices of invasive but ineffective medical therapies rather than perhaps more appropriate supportive care (Lamont & Christakis, 2001, p. 1096). Prognoses were more likely to favor no disclosure, rather than frank ones. Further, they would provide no estimate, a conscious overestimate, or a conscious underestimate 63 percent of the time:

> The fact that the formulated and communicated prognoses differ further supports the contention that these are distinct behaviors of physicians

caring for patients near the end of life, that both are (independently) prone to error, and that both are relevant to the care patients might receive.

(Lamont & Christakis, 2001, p. 1102)

Focus group studies reported that doctors expressed difficulty discussing end-of-life issues with patients with multiple co-morbidities (MCMs) as opposed to those with a terminal diagnosis (Schonfeld et al., 2012). The latter group, particularly those diagnosed with cancer, are able to provide statistics and a more complete timeline of the illness; patients and families accept that a cancer diagnosis is terminal whereas other diagnoses (renal or congestive heart failure) often bear the hope for a cure. Physicians also feel that there is no right time to initiate end-of-life conversations with their patients; however a physician may sense the need to broach the subject when "a patient's wishes seem to contradict medical reality" (p. 264). Physicians have distinct approaches to end-of-life discussions with patients with multiple co-morbidities: a direct, an indirect, and a collaborative approach, in which a specific time and place is set for the conversation to be held.

Bernacki and Block (2014) conducted a narrative study focused on the impact on the outcomes of communication about serious illness care planning, which included goals of care, advance care planning and end-of-life discussions for patients with serious illness. Consistently, a large body of research showed deficiencies in patient, physician, and systems factors in serious illness care communications. Discussing and communicating the realities and the goals of care of serious illness is a key provision of quality end-of-life care, so that the clinician may align the care provided with the patient's goals of care. Such discussions ought to be held early in the course of illness and offer "reduced use of nonbeneficial medical care near death, enhanced goal-consistent care, positive family outcomes, and reduced cost" (Bernacki & Block, 2014, p. E1, p. E6). When such conversations occur late in the illness, their impact on care processes is reduced. Systematizing goals of care include discussing the following: "sharing prognostic information, eliciting decision-making preferences, understanding fears and goals, exploring views on trade-offs and impaired function, and wishes for family involvement" (p. E1), each of them a part of attaining a good death. Discussing these goals have been shown not to incur anxiety, depression, or hopelessness in patients/caregivers as once thought and supports the illness trajectory in benefit of the patient/family.

A large prospective, longitudinal cohort study conducted from 2002 to 2008 provided important evidence about the associations amongst end-of-life decisions, patient mental health, medical care near death, and caregiver bereavement adjustment (Wright et al., 2008). Patient/caregiver/physician end-of-life discussions were shown to not be associated with patients feeling depressed, sad, terrified, worried, or meeting *DSM-IV* criteria for a mental disorder. Patients who reported engaging in these conversations were significantly more likely to accept that their illness was terminal, to prefer medical treatment focused on relieving pain and discomfort over life-extending therapies, and to have completed a do-not-resuscitate order. Patients who reported having end-of-life conversations with their physicians at baseline received significantly fewer aggressive medical interventions near death, were less likely to receive mechanical ventilation, to undergo resuscitation or to be admitted to the intensive care unit and were also more likely to be enrolled in outpatient hospice for more than a week. Patients who received aggressive medical interventions had worse quality of life in the final week of life, and quality of life decreased with increasing numbers of aggressive medical therapies. Patients' quality of life improved the longer they were enrolled in hospice, except for patients who received less than a week of hospice services. Caregivers of patients who received any aggressive care were at higher risk for developing a major depressive disorder, experiencing regret, feeling unprepared for the patient's death, and had worse quality of life outcomes compared with caregivers of patients who did not receive aggressive care (p. 1668). Such results indicate the importance of end-of-life decision-making discussions as having cascading benefits for patients and their caregivers (p. 1670) and by extension, being crucial in the provision of a good death.

A 2010 multi-institutional longitudinal investigation of patients with advanced cancer and their primary (unpaid) caregivers (Mack et al., 2010) described 325 patients recruited between October 2002 and September 2007. The patients self-reported treatment preferences by choosing either life-extending care or symptom-directed care. Those who opted for life-extending care did not live longer than those who had chosen symptom-directed care, and in comparison, suffered greater psychological and physical distress and poorer quality of life. Physical distress was lowest amongst those patients who were treated with symptom-directed care. More than two-thirds of the patients participating in the study received end-of-life care that reflected their previously stated preferences, were likely to be aware they were terminally ill, and to have had the opportunity to communicate their wishes to a physician. Roughly a third of patients who had opted for symptom-directed care received life-extending care, contrary to their wishes (p. 1206). Such data seem to illustrate that "attainment of one's goals for EOL [end-of-life] care may therefore be an important outcome of EOL care, whether goals involve life-prolonging or symptom-directed care" (p. 1203). Likewise, a disproportionate share of the cost of medical care is spent during the end-of-life (EOL), largely on life-sustaining care (Zhang et al., 2002). This observational study showed that those patients who had EOL discussions with the doctors had lower medical costs in the final weeks of life, largely a function of their more limited use of intensive interventions. The study also showed that "life-sustaining care is associated with worse quality of death at the EOL" (p. 485).

The amazing achievements of biotechnology and medicine in diagnosing and treating illness cannot alone help a patient struggle with ill health and impending death. In order to accomplish effective practice in end-of-life care particularly, a clinician needs to be competent in "narrative medicine" as well, to have "the ability to acknowledge, absorb, interpret, and act on the stories and plights of their patients" (Charon, 2001, p. 1897). With such ability, the physician is moved to absorb the narrative realities of their patients, honor their meanings, and then be moved to act in their behalf. In these scenarios, narrative knowledge encompasses a patient's personal human experiences and creates a bridge to the logico-scientific knowledge of the physician, establishing a crucial therapeutic alliance (Charon, 2001, pp. 1898–9). Without such an authentic engagement, the patient might not tell the whole story, ask the frightening questions, and not feel heard, leading to a more expensive, less effectual diagnosis, a search for a second opinion, noncompliance, and a less effective therapeutic relationship, and eventually not a sought-after good death.

A study by Johnson et al. (2000) relates the use of therapeutic narrative within the ICU to help obtain a good death. The building of narratives is employed to benefit and facilitate family decision making regarding the need for withdrawal or withholding of life support. Using the narrative to frame with words the futility of continuing the life support, the decision may be made in the voice of the incapacitated patient, by the family. In that way, technology and treatment become the villains that stand in the way of the desired result: a good death. The narrative created provides a sense of closure in that obstacles have been overcome and a good death has been achieved.

Attaining one's goals of care at the end of life—a good death—clearly is an important marker of quality end-of-life care. Communication amongst the parties involved in care goes a long way to smooth the road between a physician's obligation of informed consent and the patient/family's rights to self-determination.

3.6 MEDICAL FUTILITY, EOL DECISION MAKING, AND ADVANCE CARE PLANNING

> Increasingly in the U.S., health care clinicians fail to recognize and accept when curative goals are no longer realistic. At this point, futile efforts at cure can fuel false hopes in patients and their loved ones. The clinician's need to be doing something may result in treatment that violates the dignity and well-being of the patient and this can lead to the patients ultimate hopelessness and despair.
>
> (Taylor, 2012, p. 626)

Critical care is delivered in a highly technical area and has a strong focus on patient recovery and cure (Coombs & Long, 2008) through the use of supporting technologic interventions. However, when such outcomes are not achievable, difficult discussions about end-of-life care management and futility of treatment must be broached amongst the patient, family caregivers, and end-of-life care teams. These discussions provoke certain tensions in clinical specialties in decision making regarding withholding or withdrawing life support and elicit differences in philosophy between doctors and nurses holding different views and competing concerns about what constitutes a good death: doctors manage prognosis and outcomes for patients with difficult disease trajectories, determine which treatments should be commenced, and identify futile treatments that should not be used; nurses operationalize those treatments, futile or otherwise, manage end-of-life care practice decisions, and often facilitate the end-of-life care process of treatment withdrawal (Coombs & Long, 2008, p. 210). Conversations about goals of care in end-of-life care must be held among the professionals on a team; then, added to the mix, is the need to communicate information to the patient or family. In the case of the futility of further treatment, the consideration of limiting or withholding treatment and transitioning to comfort care highlights the need for effective use of narrative in medicine to enable a therapeutic environment and to achieve a good death.

The Problem of Medical Futility

> The simple view is that medicine exists to fight death and disease, and that is, of course, its most basic task. Death is the enemy. But the enemy has superior forces. Eventually, it wins.
>
> (Gawande, 2014a, p. 187)

Futility, from the Latin *futilis*, meaning leaky, is a concept whose meanings and implications have been bandied about since before 1990 and continues into the present. However, there is a long-standing maxim that futile treatments are not obligatory (Schneiderman et al., 1990). In 1990, Schneiderman proposed the following definition of futility: any effort to achieve a result that is possible but that reasoning or experience suggests is highly improbable and cannot be systematically produced (Schneiderman et al., 1990, p. 949). In other words, Schneiderman defined futility as an action that is unable to achieve the goals of that action, no matter how many times it is repeated. Schneiderman turned his thinking on futility towards professional standards of care, claiming that patients are not entitled to receive any treatments they ask for, that physicians are only obligated to offer treatments that are consistent with professional standards of care and are not obligated to produce miracles (Schneiderman, 2011). Schneiderman and other proponents viewed a doctor's duty as being sufficiently bold and courageous enough to deliver appropriate care to patients, including saying no to specific, futile demands and options of care. In this case, appropriate care may indicate an appropriate and good death, free of pain and prolonged suffering.

Should the potential for recovery exist, a clinician should allow for it; however, the potential for futile interventions must equally be recognized. A physician assessment of futility means that the patient will not recover, will not receive benefit from any further treatment, and that no technology would restore function. The issue surrounding whether or not physicians should be able to refuse demands for futile treatment of critically ill patients stands in direct opposition to the first principle of biomedical ethics: autonomy. Patient autonomy includes the right to be fully informed of all medical decisions and the right to refuse unwanted, recommended, or lifesaving care. In discussing end-of-life care with patients/families, "physicians should be open to dissent, push back, and disagreement, but making an expert view known is part of patient advocacy" (Caplan, 2012, p. 1041), ready to encounter autonomy (a right) and hope (a wish) as opposed to expert, experienced assessment versus inhumane, futile, painful, and costly life-prolonging treatments that are against all standards of a good death.

Advance Care Planning: The Conversation in Benefit of a Good Death

Advance care planning (ACP) is a means of extending patients autonomy to later life when they may become incapable of making desired treatment decisions. ACP is the process of discussing and recording patient preferences concerning goals of care for patients who may lose capacity or communication ability in the future, in order to improve end-of-life care. ACP focuses primarily on planning for the possibility of decisional incapacity, but it may also serve as a basis for decision making in patients who retain capacity (Tulsky, 2005, p. 360; Carr & Moorman, 2009).

Vig et al.'s (2002) descriptive study with interviews of nonterminal elderly individuals with heart disease or cancer was remarkable because of the lack of heterogeneity in the participants' responses, but it also spoke to the need for ACP, early and often. People who are not actively dying and retain capacity may express their views on their end-of-life care preferences and fine-tune them over the course of time. For providers and families, understanding a patient's wishes facilitates a smooth transition from curative to palliative care and offers an opportunity to reach consensus about strategies and goals of care. To achieve quality end-of-life care consistent with the preferences of ill older adults, families and caregivers must understand their specific wishes and general values, as well as the reasons for them (Vig et al., 2002, p. 1547).

ACP comprises a number of written documents and advance directives, such as Do-Not-Resuscitate (DNR) orders, Do-Not-Hospitalize (DNH) orders, Living Wills, and Durable Powers of Attorney. Also, various social interventions have been implemented and studied, such as "Let Me Decide advance directive programme, the Respecting Choices Programme, the Physician Orders for Life-Sustaining Treatment (POLST) Program, the Let Me

Talk Programme, the Making Advance Care Planning a Priority (MAPP) Programme" and a number of self-developed interventions such as conversations with a trained care planning mediator, a social work intervention, an advance directive tool, and a pathway tool for present and advance directives (Brinkman-Stoppelenburg et al., 2014, p. 20).

The Institute of Medicine (IOM) in its recent report (2014) favors the use of mediators or social workers in collecting ACP information (expressed by report authors during an IOM webinar, Nov. 10, 2014). In their March 20, 2015, National Action Conference (Policies and Payment Systems to Improve End-of-Life Care), speakers advocated a "welcome to Medicare" talk upon citizens' enrollment in Medicare to introduce ACP.

ACP has been shown to improve compliance with patients' end-of-life wishes and patients' and their families' satisfaction with care, and that it reduces family stress, anxiety, and depression, a big step forward from SUPPORT. However, ACP provisions often prove to be sufficiently unspecific or not suitable to the eventuality of the clinical situation of the patient, unless they are revised periodically (Tulsky, 2005, p. 360). In their extensive literature review study investigating the effects of ACP on end-of-life care, Brinkman-Stoppelenburg et al. (2014), found that DNR orders reduced incidences of cardiopulmonary support and of hospitalizations in favor of hospice care; DNH orders have almost invariably been associated with a reduced number of hospitalizations and an increased use of hospices; and written advance directives were shown to be related to an increased frequency in out-of-hospital care that were focused on provision of increased comfort care as opposed to prolongation of life (p. 21).

In a few studies reviewed, psychosocial measures were positively affected by ACP. In a sociological study, participants were found to prefer withholding rather than continuing treatment and that direct experience with end-of-life issues, expectations about one's lifespan, and religious affiliation were the most powerful correlates of one's preferences (Carr & Moorman, 2009, p. 774).

Currently, ACP is seen as most effective when used "as a process of communication between patients and professional caregivers" such as the Respecting Choices Programme, which showed an increase in compliance with end-of-life wishes and satisfaction with quality of death. These programs involve a coordinated approach to ACP whereby trained nonmedical facilitators, in collaboration with treating physicians, assist patients and their families to reflect on the patient's goals, values, and beliefs, and to discuss and document their future choices about healthcare (Brinkman-Stoppelenburg et al., 2014, p. 21).

The 2014 IOM report on *Dying in America* revealed the following findings on alignment of care *received* with the care patients *desired*. A large majority of ill adults facing end of life, those in nursing homes and/or hospital, are incapable of making informed treatment decisions, even though such patients will receive acute care from hospital clinicians who do not know them or their preferences for end-of-life treatment. Therefore, participating in ACP ensures that the goals, values, and preferences for care, when they are unable to express them, will be in patient records. Patient preferences for comfort care as opposed to acute care are more likely to prevail if recorded by ACP. People who have had conversations about their preferences, goals, and values are less likely to receive unwanted treatment (IOM, 2014) and instead are more likely to die the good death they prefer.

A prospective randomized controlled trial tested the viability of a CPR and intubation video as a decision support tool for seriously ill hospitalized patients (El-Jawahri et al., 2015). The trial included the use of video tools in a real-time healthcare setting. Patients' preferences for CPR and intubation were assessed with a baseline questionnaire, which was administered both before and following the viewing of a three-minute digital video. On the video were images of simulated CPR and intubation on a mannequin, and a patient receiving mechanical ventilation. The proportion of participants in the intervention and control arms wanting to forgo CPR and intubation was similar at baseline; however, after viewing the video, participants in the intervention arm were more likely not to want CPR (64 percent vs. 32 percent, $p < 0.0001$) and intubation (72 percent vs. 43 percent, $p < 0.0001$) versus the control participants. The study showed that such patients were more likely to not want these treatments; to be better informed about their options; to have orders in place to forgo CPR/intubation; and to discuss their preferences with providers. Such empirical evidence bears out the importance of ACP, shared decision making, and patient-centered end-of-life care to achieve a good death.

3.7 PREPARING FOR END OF LIFE: OUTCOMES RESEARCH PROMOTING A GOOD DEATH

> Dying should be as natural an experience as birth. It should be a meaningful experience for dying persons, a time when they find meaning in their suffering.
>
> (Puchalski, 2002, p. 289)

Psychosocial concerns began to come into prominence in clinical research after the SUPPORT study. Researchers began to investigate what factors were important to patients, families, and caregivers at the end of life. In an attempt to identify empirical support for the notion of a good death that might structure and improve end-of-life care and preparation for the end of life, three studies, considered hallmarks over the years, were performed by Steinhauser et al. to explore the nature of preparations for the end of life. These studies were designed using focus groups and in-depth interviews, compared the perspectives of different groups of people, and included cross-sectional stratified random national surveys. The data from these studies show broad consensus for individuals' desires in preparation for end of life "and may signal a realignment of the ways Americans view death and want to shape the end of their lives" (Steinhauser et al., 2001, p. 736).

In the first study, "In Search of a Good Death: Observations of Patients, Families, and Providers" (Steinhauser, Clipp, et al., 2000), the researchers sought to identify empirical evidence defining what patients, families, and healthcare practitioners viewed as important at the end of life, in order to improve care of dying patients and, potentially, to provide a good death. The results revealed strong agreement and variation among end-of-life care participants' definitions of good death: *pain and symptom management*, current pain control, and control of future symptoms (p. 827), was overwhelmingly the number one consideration of all participants. Participants felt that fear of pain and inadequate symptom management could be reduced by *clear decision making and communication with providers*, and felt empowered by participation in treatment decisions. The participants therefore expressed a need for *greater preparation for the end of life* in terms of knowing what they could expect during the course of their illness and planning ahead for the events following their own deaths. The importance of *completion*, of spirituality and meaningfulness at the end of life, were confirmed and participants noted the importance of life review, resolution of conflicts, spending time with family and friends, and of saying goodbye. Participants mentioned the need to allow terminally ill patients to *contribute to the well-being of others*, in the form of gifts, time, or knowledge (p. 828). *Affirmation of the whole person* by empathic providers was of importance to the patient and to the family regarding those who did not treat their loved one as their disease, and to the providers who focused on their personal relationships with the patient and family. Professional role distinctions appeared when physicians used more medical language during the focus group sessions, but all six themes were present in patient, family, and non-physician healthcare provider focus groups (p. 829).

The second study of the group, "Factors Considered Important at the End of Life by Patients, Family, Physicians, and Other Care Providers" (Steinhauser, Christakis, et al., 2000), investigated the important attributes of preparation for the end of life in hopes of assisting providers in guiding patients through this challenging and uncertain period. The survey asked participants to rate 44 attributes of experience at the end of life that had been generated by the 12 previously conducted focus groups from the first study, "In Search of a Good Death", in which participants were asked to identify attributes of a good death. As in the prior study, participants agreed upon the importance of pain and symptom management, the importance to prepare for the end of life and, therefore, of prognostication in clinical practice. Participants held a strong preference for the opportunity to gain a sense of completion in their lives and for maintaining good relationships among patients and healthcare professionals. Challenges to a comprehensive view of end-of-life care were shown in patients' desire to be mentally aware as opposed to physicians' proclivity to relieve pain. As in the prior study, the importance of spirituality, coming to peace with God and praying, as well as the importance to patients of contributing to others, were rated highly. Serving as a reminder of that no one single good death exists are four critical issues raised in this survey: African-Americans had higher odds than Whites of wanting all available treatments; participants revealed broad variation in their need to control time and place of death, with those bearing less religiosity wanting more control, and fewer than half of the sample in favor of dying at home; physicians, other care providers, and bereaved family members were as likely as females and those with religiosity to want to speak about the meaning of death.

Steinhauser et al. (2001) conducted a third study, "Preparing for the End of Life: Preferences of Patients, Families, Physicians, and Other Care Providers", that included patients, families, physicians, and non-physician providers, focusing on the questions of end-of-life preparation and completion. The study was performed in order to gain a perspective on what patients consider important to know in preparing for the end of life and how their perspectives differ from those of their physicians and family members. All study participants agreed on the importance of preparation for end of life, as well as on five other measures: naming someone to make decisions, knowing what to expect about one's physical condition, having financial affairs in order, having treatment preferences in writing, and knowing that one's physician is comfortable talking about death and dying (p. 730). Broad variation on the remaining components was significant. Participants stated that if they had time for preparation they would also engage in completion and closure, particularly: saying goodbye, sharing time with close friends, resolving unfinished business, and remembering personal accomplishments.

Other studies on end-of-life care outcomes also confirmed the importance of aspects of quality of care at the end of life:

A study to determine a conceptual framework for quality end-of-life care was performed that identified and described five quality end-of-life care domains from the perspective of patients (Singer et al., 1999, p. 164): receiving adequate pain and symptom management; avoiding inappropriate prolongation of dying; achieving a sense of control over end-of-life care decisions; relieving burden on family members/caregivers (of physical care, of witnessing death, of substituting decision making for life-sustaining treatments); and strengthening relationships with loved ones.

A 2007 qualitative study of the perceptions of persons 80–89 years old, living at home, and regarding end-of-life issues, revealed that common fears focused on the mode of death rather than the fear of death itself (Lloyd-Williams et al., 2007). A sudden debilitating disease that would leave them dependent was more of a concern than the resulting quality of life. While they did not want to leave their home, many feared dying suddenly and not being found. Many of these patients had the belief that "hospice care was for younger patients and that if cancer was diagnosed, they would be unlikely to access hospice services" (p. 63). The study subjects were aware that death could come at any time and therefore many had made plans for their funerals, had written do-not-resuscitate orders (DNRs), and had arranged for disposing the collected possessions of their lifetime (p. 63).

An exploratory study showed how elderly patients near the end of life feel about making decisions either to prolong their lives or to opt for death (Winter et al., 2007). Death without antibiotics was considered the worst dying experience, the most painful, and of the longest duration. Nearly all participants thought death without CPR (cardiac pulmonary resuscitation) would be terrible. Respondents did not know about palliative care and felt that "death would be lonely without active treatment" (p. 625). Respondents did not mention the option of palliative care until asked about it, then expressing that they felt it would be very beneficial. Most believed that death would be very lonely in the absence of treatment and often found that a reason to continue treatments, in order to have more contact with those administering it. This concept matched those in two Steinhauser et al. studies in which "participants revealed social interaction" as one of the most important features of a good death (Winter, 2007, p. 626).

A contrasting point of view of preparing for a good death came from staff, caregivers, and elderly individuals in long-term care (LTC) facilities. This point of view revealed agreement among participants on the qualities of comfort, dignity, and closure, plus sub-themes of symptom management, circumstances of death, preparation, spirituality, dignity, and lack of family burden, a motivation for initially moving into an LTC (Munn et al., 2008). The normalcy of dying in an LTC was cited as residents became "accidental witnesses to the deaths of others and described direct involvement, voluntary or involuntary, in these occurrences" (p. 489). This factor led to many residents establishing relationships with various staff upon whom they could call in times of difficulty. Hospice care was seen as contributing to end-of-life care in all ways. The central category to all the themes is a sense of closeness, because residents living in LTC and the staff working there exist in close physical proximity to one another.

The burden of terminal illness placed on patients and caregivers imposes economic and psychosocial tolls. Terminally ill patients have high unmet needs for homemaking assistance, transportation, and nursing and personal care (Emanuel et al., 2000). Caregivers of dying patients suffer psychosocial stresses such as depression because of the need to provide substantial assistance to these patients. A sidebar of the data in this study indicated that physicians can reduce a caregiver's depression simply by listening well. Emanuel et al. (2000) found that "the underlying factors that are associated with significant care needs and economic burdens . . .—older age, low income, poor physical function, and incontinence—are not readily modifiable or amenable to medical interventions" (p. 457). The best way to provide assistance to this population without raising costs may be additional hospice or home care.

Elderly patients know that they will die and claim that they would not fear it if they could know what to expect. They would like to avoid dying in pain, to die at home, to be viewed as persons rather than as their diagnoses, and not to be dependent, or a burden, upon their families. These clear and specific concerns range beyond the biomedical and highlight the added burden a doctor bears in caring for the terminally ill. A physician's focus is biomedical, but doctors also must understand the importance to patients and caregivers of the spiritual and psychosocial aspects of meaning: "at the very moment we enhance attention to the patients physiological needs, we isolate the patient psychologically and socially" (Feifel, 1977a, 1977b, p. 7). Therefore, a sole definition of a good death is not possible because people and their needs are so specific. The burden of response to their patients entails that doctors "should recognize patients' other needs and facilitate means for them to be addressed" (Steinhauser, Christakis, et al., 2000, p. 2481).

Many patients acknowledge concerns about preparation for the end of life, particularly in relation to their families. In a study of preparation for end of life in cancer patients (Wentlandt et al., 2011), better end-of-life preparation was associated with better open clinician–patient communication, as well as with older patient age, living alone, less symptom burden (particularly pain, anxiety and depression), and better spiritual well-being (p. 871). Increased spiritual well-being was also associated for better preparedness for the end of life. Increased symptom burden—pain, anxiety, depression—was negatively associated with preparedness.

From this brief sampling of the literature on outcomes research of preparing for a good death, we may assume that obtaining one has become, in the first decades of the 21st century, more of an effort to optimize the quality of end-of-life care with sound clinical assessments and by measuring the quality of dying.

3.8 QUALITY OF LIFE, QUALITY OF DYING AND DEATH, AND THE GOOD DEATH

> Quality of life always matters to the patient. Therefore, health care providers must always be concerned with the impact of their ministrations on the quality of life in addition to the effect on the disease. The recent inclusion of quality of life measurement in oncologic clinical trials research has arisen in response to a recognized need to adopt a broader mandate, that is, the alleviation of suffering, rather than the narrower goal of fighting disease. Patients, rather than diseases, are treated.
>
> (Cohen et al., 1996, p. 576)

S. Robin Cohen and Balfour M. Mount of the Palliative Care Service of the Royal Victoria Hospital framed the why and wherefore of quality of life research that became an important instrument for measuring existential well-being, in addition to physical, emotional, and support factors, in the measurement of the quality of life at the end of life.

The differences and similarities among the concepts of quality of life at the end of life, quality of care at the end of life, and quality of dying are closely related to one another and often promote confusion in end-of-life literature. Kellehear (2014–15) insisted on the qualification that "dying is living. The dying are not the dead" (p. 53). The term "quality of life" refers to an individual's personal assessment of subjective well-being (Mount et al., 2007). Many researchers have studied the factors involved in patients' quality of life at the end of life, quality of medical care at the end of life, quality of dying and death, and quality of caregivers' experience. Measuring each independently are major steps in end-of-life research in identifying the determinants of a good dying experience, towards providing a good death (Downey et al., 2009).

Because the majority of terminal patients die in hospital or in nursing homes, and because economic pressure on these organizations is high, the importance of documenting the quality of care and the quality of life experiences actually delivered to patients and their families at the end of life is important in establishing accountability. This information can assist investigators in comparing "outcomes across settings (e.g., home versus hospital) . . . alternative approaches to end-of-life care (e.g., hospice versus traditional care), and . . . care given by different types of providers (e.g., primary care versus palliative care specialists)" (Stewart et al., 1999, p. 93).

The term "quality of life", a subjective, patient-centered outcomes measure, may be defined by the physical, psychological, social, and spiritual domains of health that are influenced by a person's experiences, beliefs, expectations, and perceptions (Stewart et al., 1999, pp. 97–8). The totality of each of these factors, called the biopsychosocial-spiritual model (see p. 81), forms an attitude toward health and a belief about one's capacity to cope, which is unique to each individual. Stewart et al. (1999) defined the quality of life of dying patients, the domain that is relevant to the definition of a good death, as the "quality of dying of the patient", a personal evaluation of the dying experience as a whole, a subjective integration of some of the ". . . distinct concepts according to one's expectations and values" (p. 104). Thus, according to this study, each dying person and their family and loved ones would likewise have their own subjective idea of a good death. Improving the quality of life at the end of life is thus a multidimensional concept that comprises a broad array of needs and is influenced by "one's interpersonal relationships, as well as personal reflections of the past, perceptions of the present, and expectations of the future" (Steinhauser et al., 2002, p. 837).

The "quality of dying", defined as a personal evaluation of the dying experience as a whole, including a subjective evaluation of concepts according to expectations and values (Patrick et al., 2001, p. 718), is a term that may be used to describe the quality of life of dying patients and is another patient-centered outcome measure. The domains of dying and death are distinct from the medical care received at the end of life and are focused on the wide diversity of individuals' experiences with dying including social and spiritual components (p. 723).

Learning the outcomes measures that constitute a good death for older people at the end of life is crucial in the development of appropriate end-of-life care (Hales et al., 2010), which then contributes to the quality of dying and death, as judged by the surviving family and caregivers. The *quality of life* at the end of life is different from the *quality of dying and death* by virtue of emphasis. The concept of quality of life includes physical, psychosocial, and spiritual domains and focuses on activities and experiences while living with a life-threatening or terminal illness, which Cohen and Mount defined as subjective well-being (Cohen et al., 1996, p. 576). The *quality of dying* emphasizes the experience of preparing for, facing, and experiencing death itself, integrating the domains of quality of life with other domains relevant to dying such as life closure, death preparation, and conditions of death. Such a definition is similar to the idea of quality of death defined by the Committee on End-of-Life Care of the Institute of Medicine (IOM, 1997) as a death that is free from avoidable distress and suffering for patients, families, and their caregivers; in general accord with the patients' and families' wishes; and reasonably consistent with clinical, cultural, and ethical standards (in Patrick et al., 2001, p. 718). Patrick et al. (2001) defined quality of dying and death, the period of time leading up to a death, as the degree to which a person's preferences for dying and the moment of death agree with observations of how the person actually died, as reported by others (Patrick et al, 2001, p. 721; Curtis et al., 2002, p. 8). These are inherently subjective factors, influenced by culture and type/stage of disease.

That patients at the end of life be free of symptoms, receive appropriate information concerning their condition, as well as respect of their privacy, are included in every model of a good death (see Chapter 7). Many outcomes research instruments have measured outcomes of studies intended to assess domains of the quality of death and dying at the end of life (Hales et al., 2010), but the most well-known instrument is the Quality of Death and Dying (QODD) questionnaire. The proposed model for evaluating the quality of dying and death uses personal preferences about the dying experience to inform evaluation of this experience by others after death (Patrick et al., 2001). The six main conceptual domains within the model that help assess the quality of the dying experience are: symptoms and personal care; treatment preferences; time with family; whole person concerns; preparation for death; moment of death; and a list 31 total subscales. Due to its comprehensiveness, the QODD domains can be seen to define the elements of a good death. The QODD total score was significantly associated with constructs related to the quality of dying and death: "death at home, less symptom burden, better symptom treatment, better communication, and higher satisfaction with care were all associated with higher QODD scores" (Curtis et al., 2002, p. 27). The QODD questionnaire provides a valid assessment for evaluating and modifying end-of-life experiences (Hales et al., 2010).

A 2009 study by Downey et al. from Seattle sought to compare and analyze the top indicators of all domains of end-of-life care studies in order to standardize outcomes measures. In the study, Steinhauser, Christakis, et al.'s (2000) set of 44 good death indicators were compared to the Seattle-area researchers set of 31 good death indicators and the top percentages were found to define the major domains underlying evaluations of the end-of-life experiences. Widespread agreement was found on the top priorities of care: (1) time with family and friends and (2) pain control. Other researchers, nationally and internationally, have also identified those two items as critically important to a good death (Downey et al., 2009, p. 185).

Other outcomes studies have been undertaken to measure various factors of quality of life, quality of life while dying and the quality of dying and death—hence, a good death. Caregivers are key stakeholders in terminal care and bereavement because they provide an important perspective on, and reliable assessment of, the quality of end-of-life (EOL) care patients receive. Caregiver experiences with the quality of EOL care also have consequences for their mental health and prove to be a risk factor for poor bereavement adjustment. Research studies have identified factors important to dying patients and their caregivers, including avoidance of prolonged death or suffering, shared decision making, communication with providers about patient wishes, awareness of prognosis, and preparation for death.

Place of death is an important measure as revealed by the statistics in Chapter 2. This measure also correlates highly with the quality of life at end of life and its importance is corroborated by a 2010 study in which patients with advanced cancer who die at home do so with a higher quality of life than do those who die in hospitals (Wright et al., 2010, p. 4462). This study is the first to reveal that caregivers of patients who die in ICUs are at heightened risk for developing PTSD and bereavement-related psychiatric illnesses than are those people whose loved ones died at home or in hospice (p. 4463). Similarly, a 2012 study of advanced cancer patients who avoid hospitalizations or ICUs, "who are less worried, who pray or meditate, who are visited by a pastor in the hospital/clinic, and who feel a therapeutic alliance with their physicians have the highest QOL at the EOL" (Zhang et al., 2012, p. 1133). A 2014 Canadian study also focused on place of death, in which nearly three-quarters of recently deceased inpatients would have preferred an out-of-hospital death; ICUs were a common, but not preferred, location of in-hospital deaths; and family satisfaction with end-of-life care was found to be strongly associated with their relative dying in their preferred location (Sadler et al., 2014, p. 4).

Directly determining a patient's preferences for end-of-life care clearly can result in care consistent with their stated preferences (Reinke et al., 2013). Instead of measuring the input of patient families and clinicians, the perspectives on the quality of life while dying of terminally ill men were investigated in a study of 26 dying men (Vig & Pearlman, 2003, 2004). These patients were aware that they were dying and accepted this, reflecting on their overall quality of life, which included the importance of family and friends, of religious and spiritual beliefs, and of aspects of good healthcare (2003, p. 1597). The men spoke of their priorities as they lived in the face of death and voiced concerns about the quality of their own dying and about burdening loved ones. Three categories constituting quality of life while dying were identified: living while dying; anticipating a transition to active dying; and receiving good healthcare. The category of living while dying involved the feeling that they were still whole people having daily plans and projects: "Continuing to engage in these activities gave a sense of meaning and normalcy to participants' lives" (Vig & Pearlman, 2003, p. 1598). Well-controlled symptoms enabled them to continue participating in their lives. Participants anticipated a transition to active dying in the near future and believed that completing preparations for death could help ensure good deaths, while dying with unfinished business would lead to a bad death. Receiving good healthcare that contributed to the quality of their present lives entailed numerous details: the competency of their doctors and their willingness to answer questions; minimal waiting time at visits; and appreciation of those men enrolled in hospice of the care of staff and volunteers (Vig & Pearlman, 2003, p. 1599).

Because no study included caregiver perception of patient suffering or of prolongation of death, a 2013 study (Higgins & Prigerson) developed and validated the Caregiver Evaluation of Quality of End-of-Life Care (CEQUEL) scale to include these dimensions of caregiver-perceived quality of EOL care. Higher CEQUEL scores were positively associated with home hospice enrollment and length of inpatient hospice enrollment, and were negatively associated with bereaved caregiver regret and with psychological trauma symptoms. CEQUEL measures aspects of the caregiver experience that are of critical import not only during the dying process but also in post-loss adjustment. "Positive associations between CEQUEL scores and patient-physician therapeutic alliance are consistent with previous research demonstrating that therapeutic alliance results in less aggressive, burdensome EOL care and improved patient mental health" (Higgins & Prigerson, 2014, p. 8). The results bear clinical implications for healthcare providers, because a "low pre-loss CEQUEL score may prompt a caregiver-team meeting in which caregiver expectations about preventing a prolonged death or mitigating perceived suffering are weighed against what is achievable, and redirection of care or reframing of caregiver interpretations are pursued as necessary" (p. 9).

A representation of priorities at the end of life was investigated by Atul Gawande in his 2014 book and excerpted into essay form in the *New York Times*. As a surgeon, often treating patients for whom he could do nothing more, Gawande was motivated to research, for three years, the issue of mortality to find out what has gone wrong with our management of it and how we could do better. He said he learned two fundamental things. First, in medicine and society, we have failed to recognize that people have priorities that they need us to serve besides just living longer. Second, the best way to learn those priorities is to ask about them. Gawande also noted that the most successful clinicians had (end-of-life) discussions with patients by asking the following questions: (1) What is their understanding of their health or condition? (2) What are their goals if their health worsens? (3) What are their fears? and (4) What are the trade-offs they are willing to make and not willing to make?

The conclusions of experts' priorities; goals of care; patient, family, and caregiver preferences; and the outcomes of clinical research all point to the same conclusions: good end-of-life care can produce good psychosocial outcomes and the circumstances of a good death.

3.9 RECOMMENDATIONS OF THE IOM'S 2014 REPORT

Since the publication in 1997 of the Institute of Medicine's (IOM) last report, *Approaching Death: Improving Care at the End of Life*, healthcare delivery for people nearing the end of life has greatly changed. The current study (IOM, 2014) intends to incorporate and to build upon the former, with five recommendations that address the needs of patients and their families, and corroborate the results of the past outcomes research studies reviewed above. The first recommendation is the delivery of person-centered, family-oriented end-of-life care, largely provided by increased use of palliative care services. The second recommendation involves the need for professional organizations and societies that establish quality standards to draft actionable and measurable standards for clinician–patient communication and advance care planning. The third recommendation involves the need for various professional credentialing bodies to establish the appropriate training, certification, and licensure requirements to strengthen the palliative care knowledge and skills of all clinicians caring for patients nearing the end of life. The fourth recommendation regards federal, state, and all other healthcare delivery programs to support the provision of the quality of care for persons nearing the end of life. Public education and engagement is the fifth and last recommendation and concerns the need for public and private individuals and organizations to engage their constituents with fact-based information on informed choice and advance care planning.

The IOM's recommendations address and provide requirements for overcoming the objections to care registered by patients and families since the end of the 20th century. Recognition of the need for healthcare delivery to be patient- and family-centered is the most prominent proposal: "Transformational change is required, building on evidence about high-quality, compassionate, and cost-effective care that is person-centered and family-oriented and available wherever patients nearing the end of life may be" (p. 102).

Specialized, interdisciplinary palliative care is recognized as an essential component of high quality end-of-life care and healthcare organizations and providers are charged with getting out this message to the public. Recommendations for achieving such transformational change can only help to provide a good death: such comprehensive care should "be seamless, high-quality, integrated, patient-centered, family-oriented, and consistently accessible around the clock"; should consider the evolving psychosocial needs of patients and families; should be delivered by professionals with appropriate expertise and training; should include information transfer across all settings; and should be consistent with patients goals, values, and informed preferences. In order to provide this comprehensive care, healthcare delivery organizations are charged with providing access for people approaching the end of life to skilled, interdisciplinary palliative care across all settings; and that this full range of "care be characterized by transparency and accountability through public reporting of aggregate quality and cost measures for all aspects of the health care system related to end-of-life care" (p. 2–45).

In sum, the authors and reviewers of this report responded to the problems of advance care planning, clinician–patient communication, physician prognosis, family/caregiver stress, unnecessary prolongation of life, and unmet pain management needs with comprehensive and actionable recommendations for quality care at the end of life and thereby the possibility of a good death.

CITATIONS: CHAPTER 3

Balducci, L. (2012). Death and dying: What the patient wants. *Annals of Oncology*, 23(Suppl. 3), iii56–iii61. http://doi.org/10.1093/annonc/mds089.

Bernacki, R.E., & Block, S.D. (2014). Communication about serious illness care goals: A review and synthesis of best practices. *JAMA Internal Medicine*, E1–E10. http://doi.org/10.1001/jamainternmed.2014.5271.

Best, M., Butow, P., & Olver, I. (2014). The doctor's role in helping dying patients with cancer achieve peace: A qualitative study. *Palliative Medicine, 28*(9), 1139–1145. http://doi.org/10.1177/0269216314536455.

Brinkman-Stoppelenburg, A., Rietjens, J.A.C., & van der Heide, A. (2014). The effects of advance care planning on end-of-life care: A systematic review. *Palliative Medicine, 20*(7), 685–695. http://doi.org/10.1177/0269216306070241.

Broom, A., & Cavanagh, J. (2010). Masculinity, moralities and being cared for: An exploration of experiences of living and dying in a hospice. *Social Science & Medicine (1982), 71*(5), 869–876. http://doi.org/10.1016/j.socscimed.2010.05.026.

Butow, P.N., Dowsett, S., Hagerty, R., & Tattersall, M.H.N. (2002). Communicating prognosis to patients with metastatic disease: What do they really want to know? *Supportive Care in Cancer: Official Journal of the Multinational Association of Supportive Care in Cancer, 10*(2), 161–168. http://doi.org/10.1007/s005200100290.

Byock, I.R. (1996). Nature of suffering and the nature of opportunity at the end-of-life. *Clinics in Geriatric Medicine, 12*(2), 237–252.

Byock, I. (2002). The meaning and value of death. *Journal of Palliative Medicine,* 5(2), 279–289.

Callahan, D. (2005). *Death: The "distinguished thing". Improving end of life care: Why has it been so difficult?* Special Report 35, no. 6, S5–S8. Retrieved from www.ncbi.nlm.nih.gov/pubmed/16468248.

Caplan, A.L. (2012). Little hope for medical futility. *Mayo Clinic Proceedings,* 87(11), 1040–1041. http://doi.org/10.1016/j.mayocp.2012.09.003.

Carr, D., & Moorman, S.M. (2009). End-of-life treatment preferences among older adults: An assessment of psychosocial influences. *Sociological Forum, 24*(4), 754–778.

Cassell, E.J. (1982). The nature of suffering and the goals of medicine. *New England Journal of Medicine, 306*(11), 639–645.

Cassell, E.J., & Rich, B.A. (2010). Intractable end-of-life suffering and the ethics of palliative sedation. *Pain Medicine, 11*, 435–438.

Charon, R. (2001). Narrative medicine: A model for empathy, reflection, profession, and trust. *JAMA, 286*(15), 1897–1902.

Cherlin, E., Fried, T., Prigerson, H.G., Schulman-Green, D., Johnson-Hurzeler, R., & Bradley, E.H. (2005). Communication between physicians and family caregivers about care at the end of life: When do discussions occur and what is said? *Journal of Palliative Medicine, 8*(6), 1176–1185. http://doi.org/10.1089/jpm.2005.8.1176.

Chochinov, H.M. (2000). Psychiatry & terminal illness. *Canadian Journal of Psychiatry, 45*, 143–150.

Chochinov, H.M., Tataryn, D.J., Wilson, K.G., Enns, M., & Lander, S. (2000). Prognostic awareness and the terminally ill. *Psychosomatics, 41*(6), 500–504. http://doi.org/10.1176/appi.psy.41.6.500.

Cohen, R., Mount, B.M., Tomas, J.J.N., & Mount, L.F. (1996). Existential well-being is an important determinant of quality of life. *Cancer, 77*, 576–586.

Coombs, M., & Long, T. (2008). Managing a good death in critical care: Can health policy help? *Nursing in Critical Care, 13*(4), 208–214. http://doi.org/10.1111/j.1478-5153.2008.00280.x.

Curtis, J.R., Patrick, D.L., Engelberg, R.A., Norris, K., Asp, C., Byock, I. (2002). A measure of the quality of dying and death: Initial validation using after-death interviews with family members. *Journal of Pain and Symptom Management, 24*(1), 17–31.

DelVecchio Good, M.-J., Gadmer, N.M., Ruopp, P., Lakoma, M., Sullivan, A.M., Redinbaugh, E., . . . Block, S.D. (2004). Narrative nuances on good and bad deaths: Internists' tales from high-technology work places. *Social Science & Medicine, 58*(5), 939–953. http://doi.org/10.1016/j.socscimed.2003.10.043.

Doka, K.J., (2010). Cancer: An historical and cultural perspective. In K.J. Doka & A.S. Tucci (Eds.), *Cancer and end-of-life care* (pp. 3–12). Washington, DC: National Hospice Foundation of America.

Downey, L., Engelberg, R.A., Curtis, J.R., Lafferty, W.E., & Patrick, D.L. (2009). Shared priorities for the end-of-life period. *Journal of Pain and Symptom Management, 37*(2), 175–188. http://doi.org/10.1016/j.jpainsymman.2008.02.012.

Economist Intelligence Unit. (2010). *The quality of death: Ranking end-of-life care across the world.* London: The Economist.

El-Jawahri, A., Mitchell, S.L., Paasche-Orlow, M.K., Temel, J.S., Jackson, V.A., Rutledge, R.R., . . . Volandes, A.E. (2015). A randomized controlled trial of a CPR and intubation video decision support tool for hospitalized patients. *Journal of General Internal Medicine, Feb 18*, ahead of print. http://doi.org/10.1007/s11606-015-3200-2.

Ellershaw, J., & Ward, C. (2003). Care of the dying patient: The last hours or days of life. *BMJ, 326*(7379), 30–34.

Emanuel, E.J., & Emanuel, L.L. (1998). The promise of a good death. *Lancet, 351* (Suppl. II), SII21–SII29. Retrieved from www.ncbi.nlm.nih.gov/pubmed/9606363.

Emanuel, E. J., Fairclough, D. L., Slutsman, J., & Emanuel L. L. (2000). Understanding economic and other burdens of terminal illness: The experience of patients and their caregivers. *Ann Intern Med., 132*, 451–459.

Farber, S. J., Egnew, T. R., Herman-Bertsch, J. L., Taylor, T. R., Guldin, G. E., (2003). Issues in end-of-life care: Patient, caregiver, and clinician perceptions. *Journal of Palliative Medicine, 6*(1), 19–31.

Feifel, H. (1977a). Death and dying in modern America. *Death Education, 1*(1), 5–14. Retrieved from www.ncbi.nlm.nih.gov/pubmed/10306651.

Feifel, H. (1977b). Death in contemporary America. In H. Feifel (Ed.), *New meanings of death* (pp. 3–12). New York: McGraw Hill & Co.

Frankel, R. M., & Quill, T. (2005). Integrating biopsychosocial and relationship-centered care into mainstream medical practice: A challenge that continues to produce positive results. *Families, Systems, & Health, 23*(4), 413–421. http://doi.org/10.1037/1091–7527.23.4.413.

Gawande, A. (2014a). *Being mortal: Medicine and what matters most in the end*. New York: Henry Holt & Co.

Gawande, A. (2014b, October 5). The best possible day. *New York Times*, Sunday Review, p. 9.

Hales, S., Zimmermann, C., & Rodin, G. (2010). The quality of dying and death: A systematic review of measures. *Palliative Medicine, 24*(2), 127–144. http://doi.org/10.1177/0269216309351783.

Higgins, P. C., & Prigerson, H. G. (2013). Caregiver evaluation of the quality of end-of-life care (CEQUEL) scale: The caregiver's perception of patient care near death. *PloS One, 8*(6), e66066. http://doi.org/10.1371/journal.pone.0066066.

Holland, J. (2001). Improving the human side of cancer care: Psycho-oncology's contribution. *Cancer Journal (Sudbury, Mass.), 7*, 458–770.

Holland, J. (2004). An international perspective on the development of psychosocial oncology: Overcoming cultural and attitudinal barriers to improve psychosocial care. *Psycho-Oncology, 13*, 445–459.

IOM (1997). *Approaching death: Improving care at the end of life*. Committee on Approaching Death: Addressing Key End-of-Life Issues. Washington, DC: The National Academies Press.

IOM (2014). *Dying in America: Improving quality & honoring individual preferences near the end of life*. Committee on Approaching Death: Addressing Key End-of-Life Issues. Washington, DC: The National Academies Press.

Jacobsen, P., Holland, J., & Steensma, D. P. (2012). Caring for the whole patient: The science of psychosocial care. *Journal of Clinical Oncology, 30*(11), 1151–1153.

Johnson, N., Cook, D., Giacomini, M., & Willms, D. (2000). Towards a "good" death: End-of-life narratives constructed in an intensive care unit. *Culture, Medicine and Psychiatry, 24*(3), 275–295. Retrieved from www.ncbi.nlm.nih.gov/pubmed/11012101.

Johnson, S. (2007). Hope in terminal illness: An evolutionary concept analysis. *International Journal of Palliative Nursing, 13*(9), 451–460.

Kaufman, S. R. (1999). The clash of meanings: Medical narrative and biographical story at life's end. *Generations, 23*(4), 77–82.

Kellehear, A. (2014–15). Is "healthy dying" a paradox? Revisiting an early Kastenbaum. *OMEGA—Journal of Death and Dying, 70*(1), 43–55.

Kennedy, C., Brooks-Young, P., Brunton Gray, C., Larkin, P., Connolly, M., Wilde-Larsson, B., . . . Chater, S. (2014). Diagnosing dying: An integrative literature review. *BMJ Supportive & Palliative Care*, published online first, 1–8. http://doi.org/10.1136/bmjspcare-2013–000621.

Lamont, E. B. (2005). A demographic and prognostic approach to defining the end of life. *Journal of Palliative Medicine, 8* (Suppl. 1), S12–S21. http://doi.org/10.1089/jpm.2005.8.s-12.

Lamont, E. B., & Christakis, D. A. (2001). Prognostic disclosure to patients with cancer near the end of life. *Annals of Internal Medicine, 134*, 1096–1105.

Lee, V., & Loiselle, C. G. (2012). The salience of existential concerns across the cancer control continuum. *Palliative & Supportive Care, 10*(2), 123–133. http://doi.org/10.1017/S1478951511000745.

Levinson, W., & Pizzo, P. A. (2011). Patient-physician communication. *JAMA, 305*(17), 1802–1803.

Lloyd-Williams, M., Kennedy, V., Sixsmith, A., & Sixsmith, J. (2007). The end of life: A qualitative study of the perceptions of people over the age of 80 on issues surrounding death and dying. *Journal of Pain and Symptom Management, 34*(1), 60–66. http://doi.org/10.1016/j.jpainsymman.2006.09.028.

Lynn, J., Teno, J. M., Phillips, R. S., Wu, A. W., Desbiens, N., Harrold, J., . . . Investigators, S. (1997). Perceptions by family members of the dying experience of older and seriously ill patients. *Annals of Internal Medicine, 126*(2), 97–106.

Mack, J. W., Nilsson, M., Balboni, T., Friedlander, R. J., Block, S. D., Trice, E., & Prigerson, H. G. (2008). Peace, Equanimity, and Acceptance in the Cancer Experience (PEACE): Validation of a scale to assess acceptance and struggle with terminal illness. *Cancer, 112*(11), 2509–2517. http://doi.org/10.1002/cncr.23476.

Mack, J. W., Weeks, J. C., Wright, A. A., Block, S. D., & Prigerson, H. G. (2010). End-of-life discussions, goal attainment, and distress at the end of life: Predictors and outcomes of receipt of care consistent with preferences. *Journal of Clinical Oncology, 28*(7), 1203–1208. http://doi.org/10.1200/JCO.2009.25.4672.

Morrison, R. S., & Meier, D. E. (2004). Palliative care. *New England Journal of Medicine, 350*, 2582–2590.

Mount, B. M., Boston, P. H., & Cohen, S. R. (2007). Healing connections: On moving from suffering to a sense of well-being. *Journal of Pain and Symptom Management, 33*(4), 372–388. http://doi.org/10.1016/j.jpainsymman.2006.09.014.

Munn, J. C., Dobbs, D., Meier, A., Williams, C. S., Biola, H., & Zimmerman, S. (2008). The end-of-life experience in long-term care: Five themes identified from focus groups with residents, family members, and staff. *The Gerontologist, 48*(4), 485–494. Retrieved from www.pubmedcentral.nih.gov/articlerender.fcgi?artid=3707944&tool=pmcentrez&rendertype=abstract.

Parker, G. D., Smith, T., Corzine, M., Mitchell, G., Schrader, S., Hayslip, B., & Fanning, L. (2012). Assessing attitudinal barriers toward end-of-life care. *The American Journal of Hospice & Palliative Care, 29*(6), 438–442. http://doi.org/10.1177/1049909111429558.

Patrick, D. L., Engelberg, R. A., & Curtis, J. R. (2001). Evaluating the quality of dying and death. *Journal of Pain and Symptom Management, 22*(3), 717–726. Retrieved from www.ncbi.nlm.nih.gov/pubmed/11532585.

Proulx, K., & Jacelon, C. (2004). Dying with dignity: The good patient versus the good death. *American Journal of Hospice & Palliative Medicine, 21*(2), 116–120. http://doi.org/10.1177/104990910402100209.

Puchalski, C. M. (2002). Spirituality and end-of-life care: A time for listening and caring. *Journal of Palliative Medicine, 5*(2), 289–294. http://doi.org/10.1089/109662102753641287.

Puchalski, C. M., & Romer, A. L. (2000). Taking a spiritual history allows clinicians to understand patients more fully. *Journal of Palliative Medicine, 3*(1), 129–137. http://doi.org/10.1089/109662103322654839.

Reinke, L. F., Uman, J., Udris, E. M., Moss, B. R., & Au, D. H. (2013). Preferences for death and dying among veterans with chronic obstructive pulmonary disease. *The American Journal of Hospice & Palliative Care, 30*(8), 768–772. http://doi.org/10.1177/1049909112471579.

Sadler, E., Hales, B., Henry, B., Xiong, W., Myers, J., Wynnychuk, L., . . . Fowler, R. (2014). Factors affecting family satisfaction with inpatient end-of-life care. *PloS One, 9*(11), 1–7. http://doi.org/10.1371/journal.pone.0110860.

Schneiderman, L. J. (2011). Defining medical futility and improving medical care. *Bioethical Inquiry, 8*, 123–131.

Schneiderman, L., Jecker, N. S., & Jonsen, A. R. (1990). Medical futility: Its meaning and ethical implications. *Annals of Internal Medicine, 112*(12), 949–954.

Schonfeld, T. L., Stevens, E. A., Lampman, M. A., & Lyons, W. L. (2012). Assessing challenges in end-of-life conversations with elderly patients with multiple morbidities. *The American Journal of Hospice & Palliative Care, 29*(4), 260–267. http://doi.org/10.1177/1049909111418778.

Schroeder, S. (1999). The legacy of SUPPORT. *Annals of Internal Medicine, 131*(10), 780–782.

Schroepfer, T. A. (2007). Critical events in the dying process: The potential for physical and psychosocial suffering. *Journal of Palliative Medicine, 10*(1), 136–147. http://doi.org/10.1089/jpm.2006.0157.

Seale, C. (2001). Sporting cancer: Struggle language in news reports of people with cancer. *Sociology of Health and Illness, 23*(3), 308–329.

Singer, P. A., Martin, D. K., & Kelner, M. (1999). Quality end-of-life care: Patient's perspectives. *JAMA, 281*(2), 163–168.

Smith, R. (2000). A good death: An important aim for health services and for us all. *BMJ, 320*(7228), 129–130.

Steinhauser, K. E., Bosworth, H. B., Clipp, E. C., McNeilly, M., Christakis, N. A., Parker, J., & Tulsky, J. A. (2002). Initial assessment of a new instrument to measure quality of life at the end of life. *Journal of Palliative Medicine, 5*(6), 829–841. http://doi.org/10.1089/10966210260499014.

Steinhauser, K. E., Christakis, N. A., Clipp, E. C., McNeilly, M., Grambow, S., Parker, J., & Tulsky, J. A. (2001). Preparing for the end of life: Preferences of patients, families, physicians, and other care providers. *Journal of Pain and Symptom Management, 22*(3), 727–737.

Steinhauser, K. E., Christakis, N. A., Clipp, E. C., McNeilly, M., McIntyre, L., & Tulsky, J. A. (2000). Factors considered important at the end of life by patients, family, physicians, and other care providers. *JAMA, 284*(19), 2476–2482. http://doi.org/10.1001/jama.284.19.2476.

Steinhauser, K. E., Clipp, E. C., McNeilly, M., Christakis, N. A., McIntyre, L. M., & Tulsky, J. A. (2000). In search of a good death: Observations of patients, families, and providers. *Annals of Internal Medicine, 132*(10), 825–832. Retrieved from www.ncbi.nlm.nih.gov/pubmed/10819707.

Stewart, A. L., Teno, J., Patrick, D. L., & Lynn, J. (1999). The concept of quality of life of dying persons in the context of health care. *Journal of Pain and Symptom Management, 17*(2), 93–108. Retrieved from www.ncbi.nlm.nih.gov/pubmed/10069149.

SUPPORT Principal Investigators (1995). A controlled trial to improve care for seriously ill hospitalized patients. *JAMA, 274*(20), 1591–1598.

Taylor, C. (2012). Rethinking hopelessness and the role of spiritual care when cure is no longer an option. *Journal of Pain and Symptom Management, 44*(4), 626–630.

Teno, J. M., Clarridge, B. R., Casey, V., Welch, L. C., Wetle, T., Shield, R., & Mor, V. (2004). Family perspectives on end-of-life care at the last place of care. *JAMA, 291*(1), 88–93. http://doi.org/10.1001/jama.291.1.88.

Teno, J. M., Field, M. J., & Byock, I. (2001). Preface: The road taken and to be traveled in improving end-of-life care. *Journal of Pain and Symptom Management, 22*(3), 713–716. Retrieved from www.ncbi.nlm.nih.gov/pubmed/11532584.

Tucci, A. S. (2010). The nature of cancer. In K. J. Doka & A. S. Tucci (Eds.), *Cancer and end-of-life care* (pp. 1–2). Washington, DC: National Hospice Foundation of America.

Tulsky, J. A. (2005). Beyond advance directives importance of communication skills at the end of life. *JAMA, 294*(3), 359–366.

Van Vliet, E. A., & Epstein, A. S. (2014). Current state of the art and science of patient-clinician communication in progressive disease: Patients' need to know and need to feel known. *Journal of Clinical Oncology, 32*(31), 3474–3478.

Vig, E. K., Davenport, N. A., & Pearlman, R. A. (2002). Good deaths, bad deaths, and preferences for the end of life: A qualitative study of geriatric outpatients. *Journal of the American Geriatrics Society, 50*(9), 1541–1548. Retrieved from www.ncbi.nlm.nih.gov/pubmed/12383152.

Vig, E. K., & Pearlman, R. A. (2003). Quality of life while dying: A qualitative study of terminally ill older men. *Journal of the American Geriatrics Society, 51,* 1595–1601.

Vig, E. K., & Pearlman, R. A. (2004). Good and bad dying from the perspective of terminally ill men. *Archives of Internal Medicine, 164*(9), 977–981. http://doi.org/10.1001/archinte.164.9.977.

Waldrop, D. P., Meeker, M. A., Kerr, C., Skretny, J., Tangeman, J., & Milch, R. (2012). The nature and timing of family-provider communication in late-stage cancer: A qualitative study of caregivers' experiences. *Journal of Pain and Symptom Management, 43*(2), 182–194. http://doi.org/10.1016/j.jpainsymman.2011.04.017.

Weisman, A. D. (1974). The realization of death. New York & London: Jason Aronson.

Wentlandt, K., Burman, D., Swami, N., Hales, S., Rydall, A., Rodin, G., . . . Zimmermann, C. (2011). Preparation for the end of life in patients with advanced cancer and association with communication with professional caregivers. *Psycho-Oncology, 876*(June 2011), 868–876. http://doi.org/10.1002/pon.1995.

Winter, L., Parker, B., & Schneider, M. (2007). Imagining the alternatives to life prolonging treatments: Elders' beliefs about the dying experience. *Death Studies, 31*(7), 619–631. http://doi.org/10.1080/07481180701405162.

Wright, A. A., Mack, J. W., Kritek, P. A., Balboni, T. A., Massaro, A. F., Matulonis, U., . . . Prigerson, H. G. (2010). Influence of patients' preferences and treatment site on cancer patients' end-of-life care. *Cancer, 116*(19), 4656–4663. http://doi.org/10.1002/cncr.25217.

Wright, A. A., Ray, A., Mack, J. W., Balboni, T., Mitchell, S. L., Jackson, V. A., . . . Prigerson, H. G. (2008). Associations between end-of-life discussions, patient mental health, medical care near death, and caregiver bereavement adjustment. *JAMA, 300*(14), 1665–1673.

Zhang, B., Nilsson, M. E., Prigerson, H. G., (2012). Factors important to patients' quality-of-life at the end-of-life. *Arch Intern Med, 172*(15), 1133–1142. http://doi.org/10.1001/archinternmed.2012.2364.Factors.

Zhang, B., Wright, A. A., Huskamp, H. A., Nilsson, M. E., Maciejewski, M. L., Earle, C. C., . . . Prigerson, H. G. (2002). Healthcare costs in the last year of life. *Arch Intern Med, 169,* 480–488.

4 The Philosophy of Hospice Care, the Practice of Palliative Medicine, and the Good Death

> To prolong life by all means available to intensive care, regardless of its quality, is not to serve health but rather to fail to balance technical possibilities with informed clinical judgment.
>
> (Saunders, 1977, p. 158)

In the 1950s, concerns arose about improving care at the end of life in both Britain and the United States. Britain's concern focused on the neglect of the dying, whereas those of the United States centered on futile treatments and suffering despite the fact of inevitable death. In the midst of these quandaries, Cicely Saunders founded the first modern hospice, St. Christopher's Hospice in Sydenham, London, in 1967 (Clark & Hart, 2002). This hospice facility accommodated 54 patients dying of cancer; two years later a home hospice program was instituted.

4.1 THE HOSPICE PHILOSOPHY OF CARE

> The hospice philosophy and focus of care involve the provision of comfort and support to terminally ill people and their families when a life-limiting illness no longer responds to cure-oriented treatment.
>
> (Waldrop & Rinfrette, 2009, p. 39)

Saunders was a nurse, social worker, and physician who bore a strong Christian faith; these facets of her personality eventually manifested themselves in the philosophy of whole person care, observing that hospice is not "the care of the dying, it is the care of the living until they happen to be dead" (Parkes, 2007, p. 2). Saunders's unique vision and innovation, the focus of which was comfort care, was of facing death in a technological age. Her concept of "total pain", which proved so important to the development of hospice and palliative care clinical practice, was formulated to include physical, psychological, social, emotional, and spiritual elements (Clark, 1999). Saunders "personified the interdisciplinary, 'whole-person', bio-psychosocial-spiritual care of the dying that was central to her philosophy" (Zimmermann, 2012, p. 222).

In 1963, Saunders was invited to the United States by Florence Wald, then Dean of Nursing at Yale, to give a series of lectures on hospice care. The visit eventually led to the formation of the first hospice in the United States, in Branford, CT. That this first hospice operated within the home reflected the importance, in the United States, placed on the desire for independence and a distrust of medical institutions, and part of "a consumer movement to take back control of various social institutions . . . including health care" (Connor, 2007, p. 90).

The common aim of all hospice programs is expressed in Weisman's (1988) concept of safe conduct: "appropriate death for patients, anticipatory grief work for survivors, and maintenance of morale for caregivers" (p. 66). Weisman (1988) believed that all hospice programs have the same central purpose: to prevent bad death and to promote better death because "prolongation of life at all costs, regardless of suffering, is clearly objectionable" (p. 65).

The Problem of Pain in the Terminally Ill and the Role of Hospice Care

New, imaginative thinking about dying promoted active rather than passive measures of taking care of dying patients until the ends of their lives, centered on concepts of dignity, spirituality, and meaning. The interdependency of physical and mental stress contributed to a new way of looking at suffering. The SUPPORT study gave a disheartening picture of the social isolation of dying patients in hospital; of dehumanized dying; and of the failure of medical technology to coexist appropriately with dignified dying (Clark & Hart, 2002). In contrast, hospice is an excellent model for managing end-of-life care and a valid alternative to futile, curative practices. In the words of Dame Saunders: "The care of the dying demands all that we can do to enable patients to *live* until they die" (1965, p. 71).

Pain began emerging as a clinical specialty, worldwide, in the late 1950s. Cicely Saunders began working in the area of pain in terminal illness at St. Joseph's hospice in Hackney, London, in 1958, carrying with her a tape recorder to capture the words of her patients as they spoke about their pain—not exactly clinical trials, but similar to the method of Elizabeth Kubler-Ross, who perched on patients beds at Montefiore Hospital in New York, interviewing patients about their experiences. Each doctor talked and listened to their patients, transforming them into clinical subjects (Clark, 1999), and formulating significant theories: Kubler-Ross on the stages of dying and Saunders on the concept of total pain, a complete theory of how care of the dying in the hospice context should proceed.

Between 1958 and 1967, in 56 written pieces, Cicely Saunders demonstrated a "growing sense of wanting better to understand the corpus of knowledge about terminal pain and pain management, in order to transform it" (Clark, 1999, p. 730). While these were accompanied only by patient narratives and case examples as opposed to references, they became prominent in nursing literature. Her careful record keeping eventually became as detailed as controlled clinical trials, and by 1965 numbered 1,100 patient interviews. Saunders rejected the view that pain was an inevitable part of cancer and maintained that pain must be prevented rather than alleviated and that a full understanding of available pain-relieving drugs and the levels of pain upon which they are effective was required to accomplish its prevention. Her conviction demonstrated that terminal pain could be defeated by medicine given regularly and routinely as the patient required.

However, Saunders's approach to the control of pain extended to the importance of attention to the pain of mental distress of her dying patients. The clinical skill of listening was aligned with the art of hearing in this hospice wherein patients' feelings were facts (Clark, 1999, p. 732). Akin to the issue of mental distress was that of how much patients should know about their conditions. Here Saunders took the view that patients ought not to be deliberately deceived, that lies intended to shield them from fear may also add to their distress. In such a way, the concept of total pain eventually expanded from physical and mental pain to include patients' aspects of spiritual and social pain, as well. Eventually, in the 1960s, there arose a broader move to individualize healthcare, by taking into account the social and personal circumstances of the patient, to view care more holistically. Saunders not only founded the modern hospice, but, importantly, turned modern medicine's "there is nothing more we can do" into palliative care's "we must think of new possibilities of doing everything" (Saunders, 1965, p. 71).

Weisman (1988) identified the success of any hospice program to be the prevention of bad death and the promotion of better death, that the "prolongation of life at all costs, regardless of suffering, is clearly objectionable" (p. 65). The importance of a hospice program is the way in which it copes with "manifold physical, psychosocial, economic, and personal problems" (p. 66) related to terminal illness, thus promoting the concept of coping and care aligned with each other. In characterizing the unique quality of hospice, Weisman described the importance of promoting "appropriate" death, the central concept that "coordinates good coping and the reality of inevitable death with comprehensive service to patients" (p. 66).

Despite the size or format of any hospice program, Weisman proposed that the common aim of all of them is "safe conduct" for all those in their care. He conceived of the concept of safe conduct as having three aims: appropriate death for patients; anticipatory grief work for the survivors; and maintenance of morale for the caregivers. The entire prerequisite for these aims is the process of coping well with problems facing patients, survivors, and staff (p. 66).

Awareness and Acceptance of Death

> Some will, perhaps, find it shocking that we should speak thus of
> accepting and preparing for death and will think that both patient
> and doctor should fight for life right to the end. Some may question
> why we should be satisfied with what sounds like such a negative
> role. Yet, I believe that to talk of accepting death when its approach
> is inevitable is not mere resignation or submission on the part of the
> patient, nor defeat or neglect on the part of the doctor; for each of
> them accepting death's coming is the very opposite of doing nothing.
>
> (Saunders, 1965, p. 71)

From the beginning of the 20th century, medical opinion held that many
patients were not aware that they were dying and often required reassur-
ance that they were not, while only the relatives were told the truth (Hinton, 1999, p. 20). Beginning in the late 1950s, patient awareness of dying
began to penetrate the barriers of "collusion" among relatives and physicians (Hinton, 1999, p. 20). Cicely Saunders reported that the "truth had
dawned on many, perhaps most" (in Hinton, 1999, p. 20) of the patients
she encountered during visits. Once recognized, the concepts of awareness
and acceptance began to be studied: by Kubler-Ross with the stage theory
of dying that concluded with acceptance, and by Glaser and Strauss, among
others.

The significance of awareness contexts and dying trajectories, and the
social process and social organization of dying and death in the modern hospital context, were first identified by Glaser and Strauss. Glaser and Strauss's
Awareness of Dying (1965) provided an important matrix to the philosophy of the hospice care of terminal patients. The concept of the "dying
trajectory" revealed an image of the good or appropriate death in which
all concerned had both the time for and quality of interactions during the
dying process to reach a state of open awareness (Hart et al., 1998). Those
concerned were able to negotiate and manage critical events that marked
changes in the dying person's status, interactions with others, and shared
awareness of his or her condition.

Glaser and Strauss's classic four-point typology of awareness contexts
(1968, pp. 50–4) helped to shape communication styles about dying at the
end of life and was derived from participant observation in hospital settings.
The four-point typology runs from the two ends of the spectrum: closed
awareness, in which knowledge of dying is hidden from the dying person,
and open awareness, in which both the dying person and the relative know
that the person is dying. Two interim positions further shape communication styles: the suspected awareness context in which the dying person sus-
pects he is dying and may try to confirm these suspicions, and the mutual
pretense context during which one or both parties pretend that they do not
know that the person is dying (1964, p. 670).

The model of "aware dying" originally presented by Glaser and Strauss contributed to the ideal of a good death by providing an idealized model of end-of-life care. Open awareness allows the patient to complete the necessary tasks of dying, such as bringing closure to relationships, reflecting on his or her life, and coping with fears and regrets. The aware patient also is charged with accepting the necessity of planning for the future and of discussing end-of-life decisions such as where to die, whether or not to resuscitate, whether or not to feed, and whether or not to hydrate. In short, awareness creates an imperative for patients to openly discuss and accept that they are dying (Zimmerman, 2012, p. 222). Awareness of dying also brings the benefit of peacefulness along with relatively low levels of psychological distress to the patient while being protective of the caregiver's mental health.

Open awareness of dying has therefore become preferable in terminal care (Seale et al., 1995) because this allows the process of planning for the end of life to proceed and offers a degree of hope that the dying process may be better controlled and timed. The results of the study presented by Seale et al. were that open awareness contexts were the most prevalent, particularly in cancer deaths, with those dying in hospices and at home more likely to be aware of their imminent death.

In a 1999 study by Hinton of the awareness and acceptance of dying of 76 cancer patients and their relatives, patients' and relatives' levels of awareness and of acceptance were positively correlated. If patients were over 70 years old, weak, unable to concentrate, or had a low quality of life index, relatives were more accepting. Pain did not increase acceptance, which was "described in terms of death's inevitability, faith and spiritual values, life's diminishing rewards, completing life, final benefits, humour, sharing" (Hinton, 1999, p. 19). The patients referred to hospice earlier showed a clearer increase in awareness than those referred later (p. 32).

In a study published as two papers, semi-structured interviews were conducted with health professionals (nurses and social workers) and patients in palliative care to elicit concepts of a good death (Low & Payne, 1996; Payne et al., 1996). In the first study, health professionals perceived a good death as being one of open awareness, in which the nurses sensitively made patients aware of the nature and prognosis of their disease, while observing the correct cultural procedures necessary; and of involving the family and enabling the patient to have as good a quality of life as possible before dying. Conversely, "not dealing with patient's fears" and a patient's "non-acceptance of death" were identified as factors related to a bad death (Low & Payne, 1996, p. 237; Masson, 2002). In the second paper (Payne et al., 1996), perceptions of good and bad deaths were likewise compared among patients and healthcare professionals. Lack of acceptance was identified as one of the characteristics of a bad death by the palliative care staff, but was not specifically mentioned by patients themselves. Conversely, "dying in one's sleep, dying quietly, with dignity, being pain free and dying suddenly" (p. 312) were identified as an element of the good death by patients but not by palliative care staff.

Zimmermann (2012) saw the acceptance of death and dying as becoming integral to the provision of palliative care: "a psychological goal for patients and families, and a central, unifying aspect of the philosophy of palliative care for health care workers" (p. 221). Acceptance was thus conceived as facilitating the provision of end-of-life care by healthcare workers, with accepting patients being easier to manage and to provide with better planned care.

Neimeyer et al. (2011) demonstrated that patients with "an internalized religious worldview" experienced greater death acceptance and lower emotional suffering. Such elevated death acceptance and lowered emotional suffering "predicted approach acceptance of impending death", even though these patients were more apt to avoid speaking about death (p. 792).

Within a complex society, the definition of a good death likewise becomes complex. McNamara & Rosenwax (2007) suggested that the traditional hospice model of a good death has become increasingly inappropriate in the climate of patient autonomy and consumer choice. Ideally, a hospice good death involves an open awareness of dying, good or open communication, a gradual acceptance of death (McNamara, 1994), and a settling of both practical and interpersonal business. In order for the social and psychological aspects of death awareness and acceptance to take place, the dying person's suffering should be reduced and he or she must be relieved of pain (Weisman, 1977). Obviously, all of the factors mentioned constitute an idealized form of dying that is premised upon a willingness to agree upon what constitutes a good death, and therefore a shared cultural understanding of dying and death (McNamara, 2004, p. 930).

A 2003 study (Christakis & Iwashyna) was prompted partly by the authors' clinical observations that patients who die a good death impose less stress on their families. Patients define a good death as being painless, anticipated, and not too burdensome on their family (Steinhauser, Christakis, et al., 2000; Steinhauser, Clipp, et al., 2000; Cagle et al., 2014) and hospice care is in fact directed at realizing such good deaths by facilitating at-home death, optimizing pain and symptom relief, and enhancing patient and family satisfaction. The potentially beneficial impact of hospice on bereaved spouses was found to be "associated with the subsequent health outcomes of bereaved spouses in that it reduces their risk of death. This impact is present in both men and women, but it is statistically significant, and possibly larger, in bereaved wives" (Christakis & Iwashyna, 2003, p. 471).

4.2 THE PHILOSOPHY OF PALLIATIVE CARE

> Palliative care does not address a specific disease and spans the period from the diagnosis of advanced disease until the end of bereavement;

this may vary from years to weeks or (rarely) days. It is not synonymous with terminal care, but encompasses it.

(Council of Europe, 2003, in Seymour, 2012, p. 9)

Defining Palliative Care

In the United States, hospice care largely is provided in the home while palliative care is a consult service generally taking place in institutions. The terms "palliative care" or "palliative medicine", with their focus on the patient/loved ones and the palliation of symptoms have, in Britain, Europe, North America, Asia, and Australia, come to replace the term "hospice". McNamara (2004), an Australian anthropologist, cites scholars who maintain that the term "hospice" had come to indicate less than optimal care (p. 938), motivating the change in terminology to "palliative care". Parkes (2007) feared that these terms "have distracted us from Cicely's recognition that the unit of care in a hospice is not the patient but the family, which includes the patient" (p. 3).

The term "palliative care", from the Latin "palliate", meaning to moderate the intensity of, was proposed by the Canadian surgeon Balfour Mount in 1974. The practice of palliative care arose from the philosophy of hospice and reflects the implementation of its philosophy, but is generally conducted in institutional settings. Mount pioneered the development of a hospital-based palliative care model. The long-awaited Institute of Medicine's (IOM) 2014 report, *Dying in America: Improving Quality and Honoring Individual Preferences Near the End of Life*, performed a content analysis of seven accepted definitions of palliative care and distilled them to the four essential attributes that define palliative care: "Palliative care provides relief from pain and other symptoms, supports quality of life, and is focused on patients with serious advanced illness and their families" (pp. 2–12). The report interprets palliative care as the main means of improving the quality of end-of-life care by honoring the preferences of seriously ill people at the end of their lives. By assisting with advance care planning, palliative care ensures that patients receive care consistent with their goals, values, and preferences, including the avoidance of unwanted, painful tests and procedures that may not be beneficial. Through palliative care, patients are able to remain in their homes and receive needed support, coordinated care, and hospice referrals. The factors that have contributed to the rise of palliative care are the increases in the numbers and needs of the terminal elderly; the recognition of the numbers and needs of family caregivers; and the greater prevalence of chronic diseases (Meier, in IOM, 2014, pp. 2–16). Palliative care usage has also risen outside inpatient institutional settings, showing that the service can enhance patient satisfaction; improve symptom control and quality of life; reduce healthcare utilization; and, in a population of lung cancer patients, lengthen survival (pp. 2–20).

Palliative care has as its mission to improve patients' quality of life, particularly of people with a terminal illness and their families, and "to systematically reintroduce the human dimensions of compassion and benevolence in the alleviation of suffering within illness" (Risse & Balboni, 2013, p. 4). Hospice care stresses cooperation among interdisciplinary teams of healthcare professionals who care for the medical and psychosocial needs of terminally ill patients and their families; provides comfort care in place of curative treatment; and aids the patient's journey at life's end in order to ensure a good quality death. Palliative care likewise incorporates each of these features and has the potential to improve quality of care and to reduce the use of healthcare services (Temel et al., 2010). Within the practice of palliative care, dying is considered a normal stage of life for patients and families. The basic tenets of this medical specialty include symptom control, psychological and spiritual well-being, and care of the family, with the goal of helping patients to die with dignity (Chochinov et al., 2004).

Palliative care is different from other medical services in that it openly acknowledges dying and does not consider dying the failure of medical care. Because prognostication can be inconsistent, the use of palliative medical interventions should be incorporated early in a patient's course of illness, even in the face of substantial uncertainty about prognosis (Carney & Meier, 2000).

As treatments have been refined and the lives of patients lengthened, the definition and role of palliation has changed into a multidisciplinary model of care for the prevention and treatment of pain, symptoms, and stress among patients and families facing serious illness. The scope of palliative medicine has expanded beyond that of cancer care, and can and should be provided together with curative treatment (Epstein & Morrison, 2012; Epstein et al., 2012; Callahan, 2009). Now patients are no longer segmented into those who are living and those who are dying. This "arbitrary dichotomy between medical care of persons who are perceived as having curable or chronic illnesses and those who are recognized as dying becomes a continuum, with palliative measures gradually taking precedence over life-prolonging efforts when death is imminent" (Carney & Meier, 2000, p. 184).

Byock (1999, 2000) observed that curative treatment and palliation were considered dichotomous concepts; instead, he offered them up as complementary concepts: instead of "either/or" he proposed "both/and". In order to have a positive effect on the quality of a patient's end-of-life care, palliative care ought to be delivered early on in the disease progression, ensuring a smooth transition from curative to palliative care. However, studies have shown that referrals to palliative care services have come very late in the course of the disease and so are often inadequate to alter the quality and delivery of care provided to patients with cancer (Temel et al., 2010). The study by Temel and her associates is a testament to the early introduction of palliative care to patients with metastatic lung cancer. Early palliative care was administered to one group and standard oncologic care to another

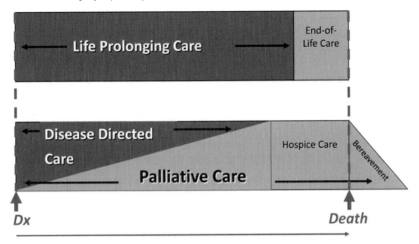

Figure 4.1   Components of Palliative Care (Epstein & Morrison, 2012, p. iii44)

Conceptual models depicting palliative care components and their relationship to cure-directed care. The top model (traditional) pits palliative care as an alternative to curative care once the latter has failed. The bottom model (new) conceptualizes palliative care as a multi-faceted palliative care paradigm involving such services early and in various critical forms, both alongside disease-directed treatments.

group. The group provided with early palliative care had a survival rate of nearly two months more than the standard care group and also achieved clinically meaningful improvement in mood and quality of life (Temel et al., 2010). The following diagram illustrates the concept.

Palliative treatment of an ill patient begins with establishing realistic and attainable goals of care, which have been elicited during patient-centered interviews. Such goals of care are important to the decision-making process because "treatments intended to cure the disease and prolong life may be more burdensome than beneficial" (Morrison & Meier, 2004, p. 2583). Likewise, the establishment of goals of care also facilitates advance care directives which then are in place even if the patient becomes cognitively disabled; likewise, these advance care directives define early on the desired quality of life the patient would want. Palliative care staff also provides coordination of an array of social, spiritual, and medical interdisciplinary care on behalf of the acutely ill patient and their families. In addition to biomedical care, palliative care also provides psychosocial, spiritual, and bereavement support to patients. If patients experience psychological distress, they may become more prone to seek a hastened death and their family members may experience more complicated grief.

The McGill Quality of Life Questionnaire (MQOL) was developed to assess quality of life (QOL) in persons with advanced illnesses and became the first study to show that hospice/palliative care can improve existential well-being, in addition to physical and psychological symptoms (L. Cohen et al., 2001). Seven themes were identified as significantly improving patients QOL in a week after admittance to a palliative care unit:

(1) changes in physical status; (2) changes in emotional status; (3) changes in interpersonal status and/or social interaction; (4) environmental impact; (5) caregiving impact; (6) changes in spiritual outlook; (7) preparing for death. The patient's comments reflect the paradoxical situation that their QOL is impacted positively by admission to a palliative care unit but impacted negatively by the progressive nature of their disease.

(L. Cohen et al., 2001, p. 366)

Evidence for Palliative Care Outcomes of Quality of Dying

Regardless of advances made in treatment, cancer remains a leading cause of death worldwide, accounting for 8.2 million deaths in 2012 (World Health Organization, 2014.) Palliative care has also been shown to improve the outcomes of the quality of dying and death in cancer care. A 2014 study (Hales et al., 2014) assessed the quality of death of patients with cancer and examined its relationship to the receipt of specialized palliative care and to place of death. Preferences for place of death always are for home deaths (Higginson et al., 2013). The study showed that the best overall quality of dying and death ratings were reported for deaths at home with home palliative care programs, compared with non-home deaths. The study also showed no significant difference between ratings of deaths in an inpatient hospice/palliative care unit/care facility and those in an acute care hospital. Late or no specialized palliative care was associated with worse death preparation, and home deaths were associated with better symptom control, death preparation, and overall quality of death.

Much important research in palliative care is undertaken in China, Taiwan, South Korea, and Japan. The cultural sticking point, however, involves the fact that elders in Asia have been typically shielded from the truth of their prognosis and impending death. However, a 2013 study refutes that claim, finding that study participants "were not distressed by the idea of death and wished to engage in end-of-life care planning so as to not be a burden on their families" (Ho et al., 2013, p. 460).

Cancer is the leading cause of death in Japan, so that the enhancement of palliative care services is a priority there. Both quantitative and qualitative studies were performed "to determine what components were considered necessary for a good death in palliative care" (Miyashita et al., 2007, p. 1090). The key components were found to be similar to those of Western studies (see Steinhauser, Christakis, et al., 2000 and Steinhauser, Clipp, et al., 2000): most Japanese patients emphasized physical, psychological, and environmental comfort, dying in a favorite place, good relationships with family and medical staff, maintaining hope and pleasure, not being a burden to others, life completion, physical and cognitive control, and being respected as an individual (Miyashita et al., 2007, p. 1094). Some other domain responses were varied, showing that, other than the core elements of a good death, no uniform styles of a good death are common in Japan. A significant difference in quality of life measures between Western and Japanese components exists in the matter of religion, an important domain in the Western studies, but not in the Japanese, possibly reflecting that Japanese do not have specific religions that are unambiguous to them. Another significant difference appears within the cultural context, in that Japanese do not want to be aware of the seriousness of their illness such that "Japanese clinicians are challenged to help their patients achieve life completion through facing mortality and respecting their value of unawareness of death" (Miyashita et al., 2007, p. 1096).

Many research studies in palliative medicine in Asia have sought to identify best practices in palliative medicine in order to improve the quality of the delivery of services. The study in Taiwan by Cheng et al. (2012) sought to identify the factors involved in improving palliative care services and formulated the good death scale, derived from Weisman's definition of good death. A cultural marker amongst Asians is the shielding of elders from the truth of their illness, such that in this study, the effective delivery of palliative care was hampered by late patient admittance into treatment. As stated by Cheng et al. (2012), "truth-telling" is the most important factor affecting the attainment of a good death (p. 854), and therefore observance of the cultural practice of withholding truth from terminal elders hinders patient autonomy inherent in communication between physicians and patients in palliative care in Taiwan.

Another observational study in Taiwan (Leung et al., 2010) was designed to evaluate the change in quality of life and the possibility of a good death for patients with terminal cancer in a hospital-based palliative care setting. As realized by Cecily Saunders, dying patients suffer from many types of loss, including physical, psychological, social, and existential/spiritual. Pain-free physical comfort is the most important need for patients with terminal cancer, followed by emotional and spiritual domains. Similar to a 2007 study by Kutner et al. that demonstrated the significance of improved psychosocial domains on the quality of dying in the face of increasing pain symptoms, Leung et al. (2010) found that "psychological well-being, social supports, and spirituality continuously improved, so that most patients could achieve a good death" (p. 1436). Such results serve to corroborate work on improving psychosocial outcomes for terminally ill cancer patients being accomplished in Asia (Miyashita), Canada (Chochinov's palliative care team), Australia (Kissane), and the United States (Breitbart, Greer).

A 2013 study in Korea (Choi et al., 2013) also sought to identify the factors associated with the quality of dying and death for patients in their

Palliative Care Units (PCUs). The findings contributed to the assessment of good death, based on the perspectives of bereaved family caregivers. Prompt symptom management was associated with PCU patients' physical and psychological comfort and improved relationship with the families (p. 740).

A population-based study in Brussels (J. Cohen et al., 2011) investigated the circumstances of death and dying of patients dying both expectedly and nonsuddenly in the Brussels metropolitan region and, second, the association between the involvement of palliative care services and the situation of the patients (p. 841). Referring to the study by Patrick et al. (2001), a high quality of dying is "free from avoidable distress and suffering, in accordance with the families' wishes and values, and reasonably consistent with clinical, cultural, and ethical standards" (J. Cohen et al., 2011, p. 840). Also, death at home is generally conceived to be a feature of a good death (Clark & Hart, 2002; Higginson et al., 2013); however, a relatively small percentage of patients died at home. Despite the suboptimal public health situation in this metropolitan region, the findings of the study supported these prior findings: suffering from cancer strongly influenced the involvement of palliative care; palliative care was also associated with an improved feeling of well-being and ease of breathing in the final 24 hours; better knowledge of preferred place of death, and therefore, an increased probability of dying at home, surrounded by loved ones at the moment of death. The presence of loved ones facilitated leave-taking, often considered a feature of good death, as it also often eases the bereavement of the next of kin.

Similar in approach to illness narratives, a research study (Yedidia & MacGregor, 2001) was designed to capture the insights of dying, palliative care patients from diverse social backgrounds in order to have relevance to a broad spectrum of circumstances. Seven motifs characterizing their perspectives on the quality of death were distilled: struggle (living and dying are difficult), dissonance (dying is not living), endurance (triumph of inner strength), coping (finding a new balance), incorporation (belief system accommodates death), quest (seeking meaning in death), and volatile (unresolved and unresigned). The personal narratives from which the motifs were assessed provide a perspective on the human experience of dying. Clinicians' understanding of them may "assist health care providers in understanding patient's preferences for treatment and their responses to providers recommendations—ultimately contributing to shared medical decision-making" (p. 817).

A small qualitative study (Gourdji et al., 2009), explored the meaning of QOL from the perspective of palliative care patients by examining patients' lived experiences and their perceptions of what contributes to their QOL. When these palliative care unit patients were asked what their ideal quality of life meant to them, they indicated being happy, healthy, without pain, and independent. These elements were all linked to each other to afford the highest quality of life to these patients in the palliative care unit.

In inpatient palliative care, seriously ill patients and their families/caregivers are the unit of care. Such patients, hospitalized in palliative care units, often have increased needs for care due to lack of decisional and communication capacity, and meeting these needs falls to the family caregivers. In a study to assess the relevant aspects of the quality of life experience for families of patients in inpatient palliative care settings (Steinhauser et al., 2014), the families confirmed the same domains and attributes of the quality of family experience previously identified (in Steinhauser et al., 2014; Steinhauser, Christakis, et al., 2000; Steinhauser, Clipp, et al., 2000): *completion*—families talked about the importance of spending time together, meaning making, sharing stories, saying important things, coming to peace, and saying goodbye, even in the case of patient non-responsiveness (Steinhauser et al., 2014, p. 4). *Symptom impact*—caregivers confirmed previously identified concerns of attending to symptoms to relieve pain, shortness of breath, anxiety, or other presenting symptoms, as well as preventing future symptom expression, and issues of dignity related to being kept clean and about physical touch (Steinhauser et al., 2014, p. 5). In both the older and current studies, the category of the *relationship with healthcare provider* produced many attributes: knowing where to get answers about what to expect about the illness, having a provider who knows the patient as a whole person, and participating in decisions about care. In the current study, families also described a desire to be kept informed in a crisis, for healthcare providers to bend the rules to accommodate family time with the patient, and to tolerate families' emotions, and to prevent problems with unclear communication by reducing medical jargon (Steinhauser et al., 2014, p. 5). Within the domain of *decision making*, families expressed the need for clear goals of care, to understand the nature of what was happening and the nature of choices, and to discuss care location choices (Steinhauser et al., 2014, p. 5). The domain of *preparation* represented the need to prepare the family spiritually and emotionally and the need to better understand the physical process of dying (Steinhauser et al., 2014, p. 5). In the original study, *affirmation* of the whole person represented knowledge of the patient as more than just his disease; in the current study the affirmation was expressed as the "ability to tell stories, participate in life review, and relay the fullness of life of the family member who in the inpatient setting may have been in a limited or unresponsive state" (Steinhauser et al., 2014, p. 6). The study participants added two additional domains specific to quality of care in the inpatient palliative care setting: *post-death care* and *supportive service*, which are not traditionally considered a part of palliative care training. These two additional domains highlight the importance of the biopsychosocial-spiritual aspects of the quality of life experience and the immense importance of the post-death phase of care for the overall experience of family members and their end-of-life memories as they moved through grief and bereavement (Steinhauser et al., 2014, p. 7).

Palliative care is also delivered in the intensive care unit (ICU). One of the unhappy conclusions of the SUPPORT study investigators in 1995 was that many patients in ICUs receive unwanted life-sustaining treatments and insufficient palliative care at the end of their lives (SUPPORT Principal Investigators, 1995). Also, nearly 30 percent of the Medicare beneficiaries in the United States are admitted to an intensive care unit (ICU) in the last phase of their lives (Teno & Connor, 2009). In a study by European and Israeli investigators, problems have been assessed with physician-related barriers for quality communication and patient- and family-centered decision making in end-of-life care that were related to physicians' knowledge, attitudes, and practices (Visser et al., 2014, p. 621). A 2010 qualitative study of patients' and families' views that helped to define necessary high quality palliative care in the ICU also centered on the importance of effective clinician communication (Nelson et al., 2010). Study participants viewed communication as promoting more efficient utilization of critical care resources by helping patients and families establish appropriate goals of care and avoid prolonged use of non-beneficial treatments. Effective physician communication was also associated with favorable patient-focused and family-focused outcomes, including satisfaction with care, psychological well-being, and consensus related to beneficial decision making. Part of the patients' and families' definition of quality palliative care in the ICU was

> . . . timely, clear, and compassionate communication by clinicians; clinical decision-making focused on patients' preferences, goals and values; patient care maintaining comfort, dignity and personhood; and family care with open access and proximity to patients, interdisciplinary support in the intensive care unit, and bereavement care for families of patients who died.
>
> (Nelson et al., 2010, p. 809).

All of these domains provide biopsychosocial support and assist in the provision of a good death.

Holistic Paradigms of Interdisciplinary Palliative Care

> Biopsychosocial thinking aims to provide a conceptual framework suitable for developing a scientific approach to what patients have to tell us about their illness experiences.
>
> (Engel, 1997, p. 523)

In the 20th century, biotechnological advances turned medicine into a cure-oriented culture with the ability to prolong life. Towards the end of the century, many healthcare professionals identified the need to balance such technological advances with a more service-oriented form of treatment, to revert to medicine as it was before modernity, when many of the nontechnical aspects of medicine were neglected (Puchalski & Romer, 2000, p. 129; Richardson, 2014). In 1977, George Engel detailed an alternative to balance the cure-oriented culture of medicine with his model of biopsychosocial care that placed the whole person at the center of both his or her psychological states and the social context of his or her surroundings. In the 1990s a movement arose in healthcare to promote what they called the "biopsychosocial-spiritual" model of healthcare, without supplying much in the way of a foundation or groundwork for the expanded model (Sulmasy, 2002).

Sulmasy (2002) posited that humans are intrinsically spiritual, based on the notion that human beings exist in relationship to things surrounding them. When humans are ill, they have a disruption of right relationships within their bodies, but nevertheless they are not their illness. Illness disturbs more than relationships inside the human organism. It disrupts families and workplaces. It shatters preexisting patterns of coping. It raises questions about one's relationship with the transcendent (p. 26). The restoration of right relationships of an ill person, then, constitutes healing, holistic healthcare, paying attention to the psychological, social, and spiritual disturbances of a person. Sulmasy (2002) called this model of optimal care the biopsychosocial-spiritual model, embellishing on Engel's notion of the biopsychosocial dimension of patient care, to describe the intersection of spirituality and healthcare at the end of life. In this model, the biological, the psychological, the social, and the spiritual are each distinct dimensions of the person, and no one aspect can be disaggregated from the whole (p. 27).

In part, the interest in a return to compassionate, spiritual care was motivated by the concept of whole-person care such as that advocated earlier on by Dame Cicely Saunders: emotional, physical, social, and spiritual. Cicely Saunders advanced the concept of total pain around which the philosophy of hospice and palliative care was organized. The term "total pain" refers to a person's emotional, spiritual, and social experiences of illness as opposed to those of only the body and its manifestation of disease (Seymour, 2012). The establishment of palliative care as a distinct medical specialty in the 1990s largely eliminated physical pain and controlled physical symptoms of suffering at the end of life. Whether in inpatient or in home care settings, palliative medicine employed an acute care model of service delivery featuring provision of social, psychological, and spiritual support to patients and their families, not simply care around the disease and its physical diagnosis. Patients were treated holistically by professional services (Kellehear, 2014–15, p. 51). Clinicians became aware that "patients must not only be made to feel more comfortable, but more broadly, provided with comfort. . . . The difference [is] between technically competent symptom management versus a holistic approach to end-of-life care—an approach that encompasses the psychosocial, existential, and spiritual aspects of the patients experience" (Chochinov, 2006, p. 84), and includes the domains of spirituality, existential well-being, and meaning and purpose.

Terminally ill patients suffer not only physical pain, but also the pain of emotional and mental distress. Clinicians face the challenge of helping patients find meaning in the midst of their suffering and chronic illness. True healing involves answers to patients' questions such as why have I become ill? What will happen to me when I die? Will my family survive my death? Will I be remembered or missed (Puchalski, 2001, 2002)? Whereas a cure may not be possible, healing—involving struggling with such profound questions with one's physicians, family, and friends—is possible (Taylor, 2012).

The Concept of Dignity in Palliative Care

> How do social forces constrain or foster dignity at the end of an individual's life? Such a question rightly concerns individual patients, their families, and decision-makers beyond the circle of immediately affected people. A society in which people die in an undignified fashion must surely be concerned with this state of affairs. And a key measure of the credibility of any health-care system is surely the respect and dignity it accords to its most vulnerable patients, those who are dying.
>
> (Christakis, 2007, p. 207)

However dignity is defined, patients who die prolonged, painful deaths, suffering unwanted, impersonal care that is inconsistent with their preferences, represent the clear definition of a breach in dignity (Kaufman, 1999). Medicine in the United States does not sanction or allow for the process of dying and physicians have difficulty diagnosing the dying phase; hence, dignity is impinged upon with life-prolonging treatments (Kaufman, 1999; Proulx, 2004). Surely, patients who die in pain are enduring an undignified, bad death while, conversely, it is undignified to deliver end-of-life care that is inconsistent with patient wishes (Christakis, 2007). Steinhauser et al.'s study revealed the desires of ill people as they confront death: to be free of pain; to not be a burden to their families; to have a doctor who listens; to die at home; to know what to expect—each of which bears a relationship to the definition of dignity (Steinhauser, Christakis, et al., 2000; Steinhauser, Clipp, et al., 2000). Sadly, the percentage of the study participants who attained their wishes is comparatively small.

As has been amply shown in many studies and articles heretofore mentioned, practitioners of modern medicine treat the disease, not the person, such that many people find treatment undignified. Deaths that occur in hospitals, apart from others, and socially sequestered, are especially considered to be bad, undignified deaths: rather, social connections are considered a key aspect of a good and dignified death (Christakis, 2007, p. 206).

In a 2014 integrative literature review, Guo and Jacelon clarified the concept of dying with dignity and synthesized common aspects of dignity in end-of-life care. They identified themes of dying with dignity as: "a human right, autonomy and independence, relieved symptom distress, respect, being human and being self, meaningful relationships, dignified treatment and care, existential satisfaction, privacy, and calm environment" (Guo & Jacelon, 2014, p. 931). The authors presented factors influencing dignity as including "demographic, illness-related, and treatment-/care-related factors, as well as communication. . . . Interventions to support dignity stressed physical, psychological, and spiritual supports not only to dying patients but also to family members" (p. 931), essentially the definition of the biopsychosocial-spiritual model of palliative care.

The Dignity Model of Palliative Care

> Because loss of dignity may enhance depression, hopelessness, and a desire for hastened death, an understanding of the relationship between dignity and these psychosocial variables is important to the overall management of terminally ill patients. . . . Whether lost dignity leads to a wish for hastened death, or merely explains the patients compromised quality of life, understanding dignity offers an opportunity to respond more sensitively and purposefully to those nearing death.
>
> (Chochinov, Hack, McClement, et al., 2002, p. 442)

Inherent in the philosophy of palliative care of dying individuals is the concept of dignity, a fundamental component of patient-centered, empathetic, quality end-of-life care. Chochinov and his palliative care research team—McClement, Kristjanson, Hassard, Harlos, and Hack—began developing the model for Dignity Therapy in the early 2000s. The concept of death with dignity in the terminally ill emerged from the ethics debate about the rights and needs of dying patients, but is invariably named in most of the literature attempting to define the good death concept. Many depressed terminally ill patients requested assistance from their doctors in order to end lives that they found medically and psychologically untenable. Concerns regarding loss of dignity were given as reasons by many physicians when they supported a patient's request for self-assisted suicide, while the same concerns were expressed by professionals on the other side of the debate. Despite the use of the term "dignity" in the patients' rights debates, the term had never before been defined from the perspective of terminally ill patients. Chochinov's team postulated that the need for skilled and sensitive end-of-life care to ensure death with dignity demanded knowledge of the concept of dignity from the terminally ill patient's perspective (Chochinov, 2000; Chochinov, Hack, Hassard, et al., 2002; Chochinov, Hack, McClement, et al., 2002; McClement et al., 2004; Hack et al., 2004).

In a cross-sectional cohort study, Chochinov, Hack, Hassard, et al. (2002) defined dignity in terms of being worthy of honor, respect and esteem. Those patients that reported a "fractured" sense of dignity reported feeling less worthy of respect and esteem (p. 2029). The patients involved in the study used their own views of dignity to respond to the qualitative study from which broad ranges of experiences are derived. Out of the teams' qualitative studies (Chochinov, 2000; Chochinov, Hack, Hassard, et al., 2002; Chochinov, Hack, McClement, et al., 2002; Chochinov et al., 2004; Hack et al., 2004; Chochinov, 2006) emerged a model of dignity that contains three major categories that refer to experiences, events, or feelings in which dignity or a lack thereof became a salient concern as the patient approached death. Each of these categories contains carefully defined themes and subthemes that formed the basis of a model of dignity amongst the dying. They help to define the concept of dignity from the point of view of elderly, terminally ill individuals and offer a model of dignity as well as a way of understanding how patients face advancing terminal illness: "Terms such as pride, self-respect, quality of life, well-being, hope and self-esteem all overlap conceptually with the term dignity" (Chochinov, Hack, McClement, et al., 2002, p. 441). Patients described situations that gave their life meaning while facing impending death, naming "essential life activities, attitudes, and self-philosophies that fostered their feelings of personal dignity; . . . life without dignity was described as a life no longer worthy of living" (p. 441). Thus, the understanding of how such patients feel offers clinicians a broader range of intervention options and provides direction about the best way of caring for the terminally ill that serves to bolster their sense of dignity, and to help promote for them a good death (Hack et al., 2004).

The first category of the Dignity Model, "illness-related concerns", derives from the illness itself as it threatens to, or actually does, encroach on the patient's sense of dignity, dictating the need for targeted management of physical and psychological concerns. Illness-related concerns such as pain were shown to be associated with depression, anxiety, mood disturbance, and psychological adaptation (Chochinov, Hack, McClement, et al., 2002, p. 441). The first of two broad themes of this category is the *level of independence*, determined by one's need to rely on others, and is characterized by two subthemes: cognitive acuity in relation to the ability to maintain one's mental capacity, and functional capacity, referring to the ability of the patient to perform activities of daily living. The second broad theme refers to *symptom distress* having to do with the uncertainties of one's health status and death anxiety, worry about the process of death and dying. The illness-related category speaks to the attentive management of psychological and physical systems because pain is positively correlated with a desire to end one's life. Therapeutic strategies may be developed that bolster independence and cognitive acuity. Specific types of psychological distress, such as death anxiety and medical uncertainty, may be sensitively managed by the provision of information about treatment options or by discussion of the anticipated unfolding of an illness and what the future may have in store (Chochinov, Hack, McClement, et al., 2002; Chochinov et al., 2004).

The second category is the "dignity-conserving repertoire", meaning the personal approaches patients use to maintain a sense of dignity. This category contains two main themes, *dignity-conserving perspectives* and *dignity-conserving practices*. The *dignity-conserving perspectives* theme relates to one's worldview or internally held qualities and consists of eight subthemes, each of which providing different approaches to assist patients retain their dignity: (1) continuity of self: the sense that one's essence continues to remain intact despite one's advancing illness; (2) role preservation: a patient's ability to continue functioning in usual roles in order to maintain a sense of dignity and congruence with prior views of the self; (3) generativity/legacy: the ways in which patients often found solace and comfort in the knowledge that, following their death, they would leave behind something transcendent of death; (4) maintaining pride: the loss of dignity in their own eyes that patients felt when they were unable to maintain their sense of pride in the face of diminishing independence; (5) maintaining hope: the feeling that one's life had meaning helped patients retain their sense of dignity; (6) autonomy/control: an internally mediated sense of self or the degree of autonomy that the patient subjectively feels; (7) acceptance: the internal process of resigning oneself regarding the changing of life circumstances; and (8) resilience/fighting spirit: the mental determination exercised by some patients in order to overcome their illness-related concerns and to optimize their quality of life. Therapeutic options relating to the dignity-conserving repertoire of this model should "reinforce a patient's self-worth by adopting a therapeutic stance that conveys steadfast respect for the patient" (Chochinov, 2002, p. 2253), with feelings and accomplishments independent of the experience of illness. Dignity is bolstered by seeing the patient as a person who deserves honor and esteem (Chochinov, Hack, McClement, et al., 2000; Chochinov et al., 2004).

Dignity-conserving practices refers to the approaches used to maintain a sense of dignity and concerns three subthemes: "Living in the moment" entails focusing on immediate issues rather than worrying about the future. "Maintaining normalcy" refers to the continuity entailed in carrying on usual routines and schedules while coping with the challenges of being ill. "Seeking spiritual comfort" means the dignity-sustaining effect when turning toward or finding solace within one's religious or spiritual beliefs (Chochinov, Hack, McClement, et al., 2002; Chochinov et al., 2004; McClement et al., 2004).

The third category is a "social dignity inventory" that represents external factors that impacts the quality of relations with others, such as the clinician supporting patients in attending to personal affairs encountered by the patient. Five themes emerged within this category: (1) *privacy boundaries* is a theme that indicates the extent to which dignity is influenced when one's personal environment is encroached upon during the course of receiving care; (2) *social support* refers to the availability of a community of friends and family; (3) *care tenor* means the attitude, either positive or negative, demonstrated by others when interacting with the patient; (4) *burden to others* denotes the distress engendered by having to rely upon others for personal care; and (5) *aftermath concerns* have to do with the distress of anticipating one's death becoming a burden to those left behind (Chochinov, Hack, McClement, et al., 2002; Chochinov et al., 2004).

One of the primary goals of palliative care is the support of both the patient and family. In palliative care, healthcare professionals support the patient and, by association, the family as well. In the model of Dignity Therapy, patients are afforded the opportunity of a type of life review, wherein they may articulate those memories that matter most to them and to discuss those things they want remembered. These discussions and recollections are recorded, transcribed, and edited into a generativity document, which is usually given to family or loved ones. This idea of generativity is derived from a tenet originally articulated by Erik Erikson concerning the satisfaction that adults may experience as a result of having generated meaningful or productive ideas and activities, such as concerns about guiding the next generation. One of the goals of Dignity Therapy is to provide patients a generativity or legacy-making opportunity that serves to decrease their sense of suffering, while bolstering their sense of meaning, purpose, dignity, and quality of life. The legacy document is bequeathed to the patient's family and often helps to ease their bereavement (McClement et al., 2007).

Such interview-based studies of terminally ill individuals reveal the importance of dignity to the experience of receiving care; of dignity as an indicator in the measurement of both physician and system responsiveness in surveys of healthcare quality; and of dignity as a key component in clinical ethics/professional practice, as included in international bioethics and biolaw (Jacobson, 2007, p. 292).

In the dignity model, empirically based on patients dying from cancer, each category, theme or subtheme offers therapeutic direction as to how to care for dying patients in ways that uphold and bolster their sense of dignity. Its importance lies in the dying patient's self-reported notion of dignity and less on interpretation and insight. "Thus, care that inherently recognises the value of individuals and tends to the patient with respect, all fall under the rubric of dignity conserving care" (Chochinov, Hack, McClement, et al., 2002, p. 442).

CITATIONS: CHAPTER 4

Byock, I. (1999). Conceptual models and the outcomes of caring. *Journal of Pain and Symptom Management, 17*(2), 83–92.

Byock, I. (2000). Completing the continuum of cancer care: Integrating life-prolongation and palliation. *CA: A Cancer Journal for Clinicians, 50*(2), 123–132. Retrieved from www.ncbi.nlm.nih.gov/pubmed/10870488.

Cagle, J.G., Pek, J., Clifford, M., Guralnik, J., & Zimmerman, S. (2014). Correlates of a good death and the impact of hospice involvement: Findings from the national survey of households affected by cancer. *Supportive Care in Cancer: Official Journal of the Multinational Association of Supportive Care in Cancer,* published online first, no. 1. http://doi.org/10.1007/s00520–014–2404-z.

Callahan, D. (2009). Death, mourning, and medical progress. *Perspectives in Biology and Medicine, 52*(1), 103–115. http://doi.org/10.1353/pbm.0.0067.

Carney, M. T., & Meier, D. E. (2000). Palliative care and end-of-life issues. *Anesthesiology Clinics of North America, 18*(1), 183–209. http://doi.org/10.1016/S0889–8537(05)70156–5.

Cheng, S.-Y., Dy, S., Hu, W.-Y., Chen, C.-Y., & Chiu, T.-Y. (2012). Factors affecting the improvement of quality of dying of terminally ill patients with cancer through palliative care: A ten-year experience. *Journal of Palliative Medicine, 15*(8), 854–862. http://doi.org/10.1089/jpm.2012.0033.

Choi, J. Y., Chang, Y. J., Song, H. Y., Jho, H. J., & Lee, M. K. (2013). Factors that affect quality of dying and death in terminal cancer patients on inpatient palliative care units: Perspectives of bereaved family caregivers. *Journal of Pain and Symptom Management, 45*(4), 735–745. http://doi.org/10.1016/j.jpainsymman.2012.04.010.

Chochinov, H. M. (2000). Psychiatry & terminal illness. *Canadian Journal of Psychiatry, 45,* 143–150.

Chochinov, H. M. (2002). Dignity-conserving care—A new model for palliative care: Helping the patient feel valued. *JAMA, 287*(17), 2253–2260. Retrieved from www.ncbi.nlm.nih.gov/pubmed/11980525.

Chochinov, H. M. (2006). Dying, dignity, and new horizons in palliative end-of-life care. *CA: A Cancer Journal for Clinicians, 56*(2), 84–103.

Chochinov, H. M., Hack, T., Hassard, T., Kristjanson, L. J., McClement, S. E., & Harlos, M. (2002). Dignity in the terminally ill: A cross-sectional, cohort study. *Lancet, 360*(9350), 2026–2030. http://doi.org/10.1016/S0140–6736(02)12022–8.

Chochinov, H. M., Hack, T., Hassard T., Kristjanson L. J., McClement, S. E., Harlos, M. (2004). Dignity and psychotherapeutic considerations in end-of-life care. *Journal of Palliative Care, 20*(3), 134–142.

Chochinov, H. M., Hack, T., McClement, S. E., Kristjanson, L., & Harlos, M. (2002). Dignity in the terminally ill: A developing empirical model. *Social Science & Medicine (1982), 54*(3), 433–443. Retrieved from www.ncbi.nlm.nih.gov/pubmed/11824919.

Christakis, N. (2007). The social origins of dignity in medical care at the end of life. In J. Malpas & N. Lickiss (Eds.), *Perspectives on human dignity: A conversation* (eBook, Vol. 284) (pp. 199–207). Dordrecht: Springer.

Christakis, N. A., & Iwashyna, T. J. (2003). The health impact of health care on families: A matched cohort study of hospice use by decedents and mortality outcomes in surviving, widowed spouses. *Social Science & Medicine, 57*(3), 465–475. Retrieved from www.ncbi.nlm.nih.gov/pubmed/12791489.

Clark, D. (1999). "Total pain," disciplinary power and the body in the work of Cicely Saunders, 1958–1967. *Social Science & Medicine, 49*(1999), 727–736.

Clark, D., & Hart, D. (2002). Between hope and acceptance: The medicalisation of dying. *BMJ, 324*(7342), 905–907.

Cohen, J., Houttekier, D., Chambaere, K., Bilsen, J., & Deliens, L. (2011). The use of palliative care services associated with better dying circumstances. Results from an epidemiological population-based study in the Brussels metropolitan region. *Journal of Pain and Symptom Management, 42*(6), 839–851. http://doi.org/10.1016/j.jpainsymman.2011.02.017.

Cohen, L. M., Poppel, D. M., Cohn, G. M., & Reiter, G. S. (2001). A very good death: Measuring quality of dying in end-stage renal disease. *Journal of Palliative Medicine, 4*(2), 167–172. Retrieved from www.ncbi.nlm.nih.gov/pubmed/11441625.

Connor, S. (2007). Development of hospice and palliative care in the United States. *OMEGA—The Journal of Death and Dying, 56*(1), 89–99. http://doi.org/10.2190/OM.56.1.h.

Engel, G. L. (1997). From biomedical to biopsychosocial. Being scientific in the human domain. *Psychosomatics, 38*(6), 521–528. http://doi.org/10.1016/S0033-3182(97)71396-3.

Epstein, A. S., Goldberg, G. R., & Meier, D. E. (2012). Palliative care and hematologic oncology: The promise of collaboration. *Blood Reviews, 26*(6), 233–239. http://doi.org/10.1016/j.blre.2012.07.001.

Epstein, A. S., & Morrison, R. S. (2012). Palliative oncology: Identity, progress, and the path ahead. *Annals of Oncology: Official Journal of the European Society for Medical Oncology/ESMO, 23*(Suppl. 3), iii43–iii48. http://doi.org/10.1093/annonc/mds087.

Glaser, B. G., & Strauss, A. S. (1964). Awareness contexts and social interaction. *American Sociological Review, 29*(5), 669–679. http://doi.org/10.1126/science.135.3503.554.

Glaser, B. G., & Strauss, A. S. (1965). *Awareness of dying.* Chicago: Aldine Publishing Co.

Glaser, B. G., & Strauss, A. G. (1968). *Time for dying.* Chicago: Aldine Publishing Company.

Gourdji, I., McVey, L., & Purden, M. (2009). A quality end of life from a palliative care patient's perspective. *Journal of Palliative Medicine, 25*(1), 40–50.

Guo, Q., & Jacelon, C. S. (2014). An integrative review of dignity in end-of-life care. *Journal of Palliative Medicine, 28*(7), 931–940. http://doi.org/10.1177/0269216314528399.

Hack, T. F., Chochinov, H. M., Hassard, T., Kristjanson, L. J., McClement, S. E., & Harlos, M. (2004). Defining dignity in terminally ill cancer patients: A factor-analytic approach. *Psycho-Oncology, 13*(10), 700–708. http://doi.org/10.1002/pon.786.

Hart, B., Sainsbury, P., & Short, S. (1998). Whose dying? A sociological critique of the "good death." *Mortality, 3*(1), 65–77. http://doi.org/10.1080/713685884.

Higginson, I. J., Sarmento, V. P., Calanzani, N., Benalia, H., & Gomes, B. (2013). Dying at home—Is it better: A narrative appraisal of the state of the science. *Journal of Palliative Medicine, 27*(10), 918–924. http://doi.org/10.1177/0269216313487940.

Hinton, J. (1999). The progress of awareness and acceptance of dying assessed in cancer patients and their caring relatives. *Journal of Palliative Medicine, 13*, 19–35.

Ho, A.H.Y., Chan, C.L.W., Leung, P.P.Y., Chochinov, H. M., Neimeyer, R. A, Pang, S.M.C., & Tse, D.M.W. (2013). Living and dying with dignity in Chinese society: Perspectives of older palliative care patients in Hong Kong. *Age and Ageing, 42*(4), 455–461. http://doi.org/10.1093/ageing/aft003.

IOM (2014).*Dying in America: Improving quality & honoring individual preferences near the end of life,* Committee on Approaching Death: Addressing Key End-of-Life Issues. Washington, DC: The National Academies Press.

Jacobson, N. (2007). Dignity and health: A review. *Social Science & Medicine (1982), 64*(2), 292–302. http://doi.org/10.1016/j.socscimed.2006.08.039.

Kaufman, S. (1999). The clash of meanings: Medical narrative and biographical story at life's end. *Generations, 23*(4), 77–82.

Kellehear, A. (2014–15). Is "healthy dying" a paradox? Revisiting an early Kastenbaum. *OMEGA—Journal of Death and Dying, 70*(1), 43–55.

Kutner, J. S., Bryant, L. L., Beaty, B. L., & Fairclough, D. L. (2007). Time course and characteristics of symptom distress and quality of life at the end of life. *Journal* of Pain and Symptom Management, 34(3), 227–236. http://doi.org/10.1016/j.jpainsymman.2006.11.016.

Leung, K., Tsai, J., Cheng, S., Liu, W., Chiu, T., Wu, C., & Chen, C. (2010). Can a good death and quality of life be achieved for patients with terminal cancer in a palliative care unit? *Journal of Palliative Medicine, 13*(12), 1433–1438. http://doi.org/10.1089/jpm.2010.0240.

Low, J.T., & Payne, S. (1996). The good and bad death perceptions of health professionals working in palliative care. *European Journal of Cancer Care, 5*(4), 237–241. Retrieved from www.ncbi.nlm.nih.gov/pubmed/9117068.

Masson, J.D. (2002). Non-professional perceptions of "good death ": A study of the views of hospice care patients and relatives of deceased hospice care patients. *Mortality, 7*(2), 191–209. http://doi.org/10.1080/1357627022013629.

McClement, S.E., Chochinov, H.M., Hack, T., Hassard, T., Kristjanson, L.J., & Harlos, M. (2007). Dignity therapy: Family member perspectives. *Journal of Palliative Medicine, 10*(5), 1076–1082. http://doi.org/10.1089/jpm.2007.0002.

McClement, S.E., Chochinov, H.M., Hack, T.F., Kristjanson, L.J., Harlos, M. (2004). Dignity conserving care: Application of research findings to practice. *International Journal of Palliative Nursing, 10*(4), 173–179.

McNamara, B. (2004). Good enough death: Autonomy and choice in Australian palliative care. *Social Science & Medicine, 58*(5), 929–938. http://doi.org/10.1016/j.socscimed.2003.10.042.

McNamara, B., & Rosenwax, L. (2007). Mismanagement of dying. *Health Sociology Review, 16*(5), 373–383.

Miyashita, M., Sanjo, M., Morita, T., Hirai, K., & Uchitomi, Y. (2007). Good death in cancer care: A nationwide quantitative study. *Annals of Oncology: Official Journal of the European Society for Medical Oncology/ESMO, 18*(6), 1090–1097. http://doi.org/10.1093/annonc/mdm068.

Morrison, R.S., & Meier, D.E. (2004). Palliative care. *New England Journal of Medicine, 350*, 2582–2590.

Neimeyer, R.A., Currier, J.M., Coleman, R., Tomer, A., & Samuel, E. (2011). Confronting suffering and death at the end of life: The impact of religiosity, psychosocial factors, and life regret among hospice patients. *Death Studies, 35*(9), 777–800. http://doi.org/10.1080/07481187.2011.583200.

Nelson, J, E, Puntillo, K.A., . . . Penrod, J. (2010). In their own words: Patients and families define high-quality palliative care in the intensive care unit. *Critical Care Medicine, 38*(3), 808–818.

Parkes, C.M., (2007). Introduction: Hospice heritage. *OMEGA—The Journal of Death and Dying, 56*(1), 1–5. http://doi.org/10.2190/OM.56.1.a.

Patrick, D.L., Engelberg, R.A., & Curtis, J.R. (2001). Evaluating the quality of dying and death. *Journal of Pain and Symptom Management, 22*(3), 717–726. Retrieved from www.ncbi.nlm.nih.gov/pubmed/11532585.

Payne, S., Langley-Evans, A., & Hillier, R. (1996). Perceptions of a "good" death: A comparative study of the views of hospice staff and patients. *Palliative Medicine, 10*(4), 307–312. http://doi.org/10.1177/026921639601000406.

Proulx, K. (2004). Dying with dignity: The good patient versus the good death. *American Journal of Hospice & Palliative Medicine, 21*(2), 116–120. http://doi.org/10.1177/104990910402100209.

Puchalski, C.M. (2001). The role of spirituality in health care. *Proceedings (Baylor University. Medical Center), 14*(4), 352–357. Retrieved from www.ncbi.nlm.nih.gov/pubmed/24041177.

Puchalski, C.M. (2002). Spirituality and end-of-life care: A time for listening and caring. *Journal of Palliative Medicine, 5*(2), 289–294. http://doi.org/10.1089/109662102753641287.

Puchalski, C. M., & Romer, A. L. (2000). Taking a spiritual history allows clinicians to understand patients more fully. *Journal of Palliative Medicine, 3*(1), 129–137. http://doi.org/10.1089/109662103322654839.

Richardson, P. (2014). Spirituality, religion and palliative care. *Annals of Palliative Medicine, 3*(3), 150–159. http://doi.org/10.3978/j.issn.2224–5820.2014.07.05.

Risse, G. B., & Balboni, M. J. (2013). Shifting hospital-hospice boundaries: Historical perspectives on the institutional care of the dying. *The American Journal of Hospice & Palliative Care, 30*(4), 325–330. http://doi.org/10.1177/1049909112452336.

Saunders, C. (1965). The last stages of life. *The American Journal of Nursing, 65*(3), 70–75.

Saunders, C. (1977). Dying they live: St. Christopher's Hospice. In H. Feifel (Ed.), *New meanings of death* (pp. 153–179). New York: McGraw Hill.

Seale, C., Addington-Hall, J., & McCarthy, M. (1995). Awareness of dying: Prevalence, causes and consequences. *Social Science & Medicine, 45*(3), 477–484. Retrieved from www.ncbi.nlm.nih.gov/pubmed/9232741.

Seymour, J. (2012). Looking back, looking forward: The evolution of palliative and end-of-life care in England. *Mortality, 17*(1), 1–18.

Steinhauser, K. E., Christakis, N. A., Clipp, E. C., McNeilly, M., McIntyre, L., & Tulsky, J. A. (2000). Factors considered important at the end of life by patients, family, physicians, and other care providers. *JAMA, 284*(19), 2476–2482. http://doi.org/10.1001/jama.284.19.2476.

Steinhauser, K. E., Clipp, E. C., McNeilly, M., Christakis, N. A, McIntyre, L. M., & Tulsky, J. A. (2000). In search of a good death: Observations of patients, families, and providers. *Annals of Internal Medicine, 132*(10), 825–832. Retrieved from http://www.ncbi.nlm.nih.gov/pubmed/10819707.

Steinhauser, K. E., Voils, C. I., Bosworth, H., & Tulsky, J. A. (2014). What constitutes quality of family experience at the end of life? Perspectives from family members of patients who died in the hospital. *Palliative & Supportive Care*, published online first, pp. 1–8. http://doi.org/10.1017/S1478951514000807.

Sulmasy, D. P. (2002). A biopsychosocial-spiritual model for the care of patients at the end of life. *The Gerontologist, 42* (Spec. No. III), 24–33. Retrieved from www.ncbi.nlm.nih.gov/pubmed/12415130.

SUPPORT Principal Investigators (1995). A controlled trial to improve care for seriously ill hospitalized patients, *JAMA, 274*(20), 1591–1598.

Taylor, C. (2012). Rethinking hopelessness and the role of spiritual care when cure is no longer an option. *Journal of Pain and Symptom Management, 44*(4), 626–630. http://doi.org/10.1016/j.jpainsymman.2012.07.010.

Temel, J. S., Greer, J. A., Muzikansky, A., Gallagher, E. R., Admane, S., Jackson, V. A., . . . Lynch, T. J. (2010). Early palliative care for patients with metastatic non-small-cell lung cancer. *The New England Journal of Medicine, 363*(8), 733–742. http://doi.org/10.1056/NEJMoa1000678.

Teno, J. M., & Connor, S. R. (2009). Referring a patient and family to high-quality palliative care at the close of life: "We met a new personality . . . with this level of compassion and empathy." *JAMA, 301*(6), 651–660.

Visser, M., Deliens, L., & Houttekier, D. (2014). Physician-related barriers to communication and patient and family-centred decision making towards the end of life in intensive care: A systematic review. *Critical Care (London, England), 18*(6), 604–623. http://doi.org/10.1186/s13054–014–0604-z.

Waldrop, D. P., & Rinfrette, E. S. (2009). Can short hospice enrollment be long enough? Comparing the perspectives of hospice professionals and family caregivers. *Palliative & Supportive Care, 7*(1), 37–47. http://doi.org/10.1017/S1478951509000066.

Weisman, A. D. (1977). The psychiatrist and the inexorable. In H. Feifel (Ed.), *New meanings of death* (pp. 107–122). New York: McGraw Hill & Co.

Weisman, A. D. (1988). Appropriate death and the hospice program. *The Hospice Journal, 41*(1), 65–77.

World Health Organization. (2014). Cancer fact sheet #297. Retrieved from www.who.int/mediacentre/factsheets/fs297/en/.

Yedidia, M. J., & MacGregor, B. (2001). Confronting the prospect of dying. Reports of terminally ill patients. *Journal of Pain and Symptom Management, 22*(4), 807–819. Retrieved from www.ncbi.nlm.nih.gov/pubmed/11576797.

Zimmermann, C. (2012). Acceptance of dying: A discourse analysis of palliative care literature. *Social Science & Medicine, 75*(1), 217–224.

Part II

Psychosocial Interventions to Promote a Good Death

Psychosocial care has been defined as "concern with the psycho-logical and emotional well-being of the patient and their family/carers, including issues of self-esteem, insight into an adaption to illness and its consequences, communication, social functioning and relationships."

(Hudson et al., 2010, p. 1).

The terminal elderly face not only the reality of their diagnosis but also cop-ing with that of aging: physical losses, comorbid medical problems, personal losses, and isolation and loneliness. Even physically healthy individuals often suffer depression and anxiety (Holland et al., 2009). Other quality of life factors facing such individuals include existential concerns, despair, and demoralization (Kissane et al., 2004). Therefore, psychiatrists, particularly within oncology, are in the vanguard of providers that have responded to these difficulties with various types of psychosocial and psychotherapeutic interventions.

This section of the book, then, will focus on the psychosocial concepts and interventions that have the potential to bolster the coping of individuals with a terminal illness facing death at the end of life: those involving spiritu-ality, hope, life review, existentialism, and meaning making.

5   The Psychosocial Viewpoint

> The psychosocial viewpoint . . . is an effort to gather more informa-
> tion about a sick patient, but in the direction of how he adapts to
> illness and maintains equilibrium in the presence of social, economic,
> emotional disruptions.
>
> (Weisman, 1974, p. 22)

The publishing of the SUPPORT study in the late 1990s "documented high
levels of untreated pain and poor communication" as well as frequent misunderstandings regarding patients' end-of-life preferences (Chibnall et al.,
2004, p. 419). Other studies confirmed that the psychosocial-spiritual needs
of patients at the end of life—including attention to the patient's emotional
state, the importance of social support and spirituality in the patient's experience of dying—are subject to similar processes of avoidance, miscom-
munication, and misunderstanding (Block, 2001). The culture of clinical
medicine that "selects and trains technically competent physicians does not
value" psychosocial-spiritual measures and so "creates a work environment
hostile" to psychosocial-spiritual concerns (Chibnall et al., 2004, p. 423).

Psychosocial factors play a major role in end-of-life (EOL) decision making. Because the majority of deaths occur after some sort of decision has
been made, such as the withholding or withdrawing of treatment, they are a
crucial aspect of providing quality EOL care. Quality of care at the end-of-
life includes the alleviation of pain and suffering, not only of the physical/
medical interventions, but also of behavioral ones. In order to relieve suffering, mental health practitioners also began to participate in the treatment of
the whole person, the biopsychosocial-spiritual being, the model of holistic
care proposed by Engel in 1977 that features patient-centered care (Frankel & Quill, 2005; Richardson, 2014).

Formerly, doctors withheld the diagnosis and prognosis of their disease
from patients, thinking to avert fear and stigma. However, in the majority of
developed countries today, patients learn their diagnosis and are informed
about their treatment options. This change permitted the first formal psychosocial studies of patients in the 1950s, and the beginning of research into

coping and development of interventions to improve quality of life (Holland, 2004). The psychosocial domain was slow to develop due to persisting attitudinal barriers that curtailed the implementation of quality psychosocial care. Holland (2010) proposed stigma as a major barrier that delayed patients' asking for help and oncologists' integrating psychosocial care into their practice. The emergence of the field of psychosocial care arose fairly recently, in the 1970s, with the lifting of two stigmas—of cancer and of mental illness/psychological difficulties—making it possible to study psychosocial issues openly (Holland, 2010; Jacobsen et al., 2012). Psychosocial care of cancer patients, and later of those with other terminal diagnoses, grew apace into the field of psycho-oncology and evolved into an important dimension of palliative care. Due to the publication in 2007 of the Institute of Medicine (IOM) report *Cancer Care for the Whole Patient: Meeting Psychosocial Health Needs*, the field of psychosocial care in oncology received increased attention. One of the report's major conclusions is that, despite good evidence for the effectiveness of psychosocial services such as counseling and psychotherapy in meeting patients' psychosocial needs, cancer care often fails to address these needs. The reasons for this failure are many and include the tendency of oncology care providers to underestimate distress in patients and to not link patients to appropriate services when needs are identified (Jacobsen, 2009)

The IOM panel found "evidence for the effectiveness of an array of formal psychosocial services including counseling and psychotherapy, pharmacologic management of mental symptoms, illness self-management and self-care programs, family and caregiver education, and health promotion interventions" (Jacobsen et al., 2012, p. 1151).

An important goal of psychosocial care is "to recognize and address the effects that cancer and its treatment have on the mental status and emotional well-being of patients, their family members, and their professional caregivers" (Jacobsen et al., 2012, p. 1151). A substantial evidence base confirms that cancer patients experience significant psychosocial symptoms. "Psychological distress, including anxiety, depression, and changes in mood, affects over 35% of all patients with cancer" (Abernethy et al., 2010, p. 894). Studies have found that depression diminishes cancer patients' quality of life and that a faster rate of disease progression and a greater severity of other cancer-related symptoms, particularly pain, are associated with depression.

Amongst the psychosocial issues for which mental health providers must assess a terminally ill patient are: the emotional burden of diagnosable mental disorders (anxiety disorders, clinical depression/other mood disorders, delirium, dementia, personality disorders, and substance abuse); intrapersonal issues (autonomy/control, dignity, decision-making capacity, existential issues, demoralization, spiritual beliefs, fear, grief/loss, and hopelessness); and the social context of interpersonal/environmental issues (being a burden, cultural factors that impact the provision of care, financial variables, and presence/absence of significant individuals, the lack of which occasions isolation/loneliness) (Werth et al., 2002, pp. 404–7; Frankel & Quill, 2005; Holland et al., 2009; Howell et al., 2012).

Psychosocial factors, such as psychological, spiritual, emotional, intellectual, interpersonal, and social issues, in addition to the medical issues of the terminally ill, play an important role in end-of-life care and are a major determinant of well-being (Baker, 2005; Rodin, 2013). Such factors relate to the broad range of human issues about the end of life including concern for loved ones, for spiritual well-being, for having the opportunity to say goodbye, and for independence and control, as well as for comfort (Bernacki & Block, 2014; Steinhauser et al., 2000). Studies have indicated that positive psychosocial intervention improves the well-being of terminally ill patients (Chow et al., 2004; Guo et al., 2013), boosting quality of life and psychological well-being. In addition to improving emotional well-being and mental health, psychosocial care has been shown to promote better management of common disease-related symptoms and adverse effects of treatment, such as pain and fatigue (Jacobsen et al., 2012).

One of the goals of palliative care is to provide psychosocial support to patients and families facing terminal illness. Early psychosocial research was conducted almost entirely to benefit elderly patients dying with chronic medical illnesses. More recent studies have focused earlier in the disease trajectory of life-threatening illness, similar to current palliative care practice as a whole. Such interventions, such as CALM, MMI, and other psychotherapy-based interventions potentially allow patients with advanced illness to continue to engage in living, while possibly transitioning from cure to care.

Currently, the primary mode of delivering psychosocial care to cancer patients is through adjunctive programs (e.g., psychotherapy, support groups, and psycho-education). These services are typically provided by social workers, counselors, and chaplains in parallel with medical care. Clinical researchers have also investigated and developed several programs for psychosocial interventions, such as: PATHFINDER (Abernethy et al., 2010); Managing Cancer and Living Meaningfully (CALM) (Nissim et al., 2012); OUTLOOK life review intervention (Steinhauser et al., 2008); Life Tape Project life review/legacy (LTP) (Garlan et al., 2010); Mindfulness Based Stress Reduction (MBSR) (Greene et al., 2012); Short-Term Life Review (Ando et al., 2010); the Meaning-Making intervention (MMi) (Lee et al., 2006; Lee, 2008); the development of a Geriatric-Specific Group Psychoeducational Intervention based on Erikson's stages of development and Folkman's model of coping (Holland et al., 2009), as well as the existential psychotherapy interventions of SEGT and CEGT (Kissane et al., 2003; Kissane et al., 2004; Kissane et al., 2007); Supportive-Affective Group Experience for Persons with Life-Threatening Illness (LTI-SAGE) (Miller et al., 2007); Living with Hope Program (LWHP) (Duggleby et al., 2007); Cognitive Behavioral Therapy (CBT) (Greer et al., 2010; Greer et al., 2012); the Meaning Making Group/Private Interventions (Breitbart et al., 2010;

Breitbart et al., 2012; Breitbart et al., 2015); and Dignity Therapy (Chochinov, 2004, 2007).

Much literature on psychosocial care of the dying has been and is still being published, but little is written about the problem of delivering this care efficiently. Research continues to identify the unmet psychosocial needs of patients along with limited service availability, service accessibility, and poor uptake of psychosocial interventions. In spite of the availability, internationally, of evidence-based clinical practice guidelines about the need to improve psychosocial care, "implementation into routine care is limited" (Dilworth et al., 2014). Dilworth et al. (2014) examined the barriers to patients and to providers. The two principal findings about overcoming these barriers to embedding psychosocial care into daily routines were the need for clear promotion of psychosocial care among patients with cancer and lack of time for clinicians to integrate psychosocial care into daily practice. The need to overcome many of the organizational, cultural, and individual barriers could be "capability building strategies, such as communications skills training, clinical supervision and interventions that clearly map care pathways" (Dilworth et al., 2014).

CITATIONS: CHAPTER 5

Abernethy, A.P., Herndon, J.E., Coan, A., Staley, T., Wheeler, J.L., Rowe, K., . . . Lyerly, H.K. (2010). Phase 2 pilot study of pathfinders: A psychosocial intervention for cancer patients. *Supportive Care in Cancer, 18*(7), 893–898. http://doi.org/10.1007/s00520-010-0823-z.

Ando, M., Morita, T., Akechi, T., & Okamoto, T. (2010). Efficacy of short-term life-review interviews on the spiritual well-being of terminally ill cancer patients. *Journal of Pain and Symptom Management, 39*(6), 993–1002. http://doi.org/10.1016/j.jpainsymman.2009.11.320.

Baker, M. (2005). Facilitating forgiveness and peaceful closure: The therapeutic value of psychosocial intervention in end-of-life care, *Journal of Social Work in End-of-Life & Palliative Care, 1*(4), 83–97. http://doi.org/10.1300/J457v01n04.

Bernacki, R.E., & Block, S.D. (2014). Communication about serious illness care goals. *JAMA Internal Medicine, 174*(12), 1994–2003. http://doi.org/10.1001/jamainternmed.2014.5271.

Block, S. (2001). Psychological considerations, growth, and transcendence at the end of life: The art of the possible. *JAMA: The Journal of the American Medical Association, 285*(22), 2898–2906. Retrieved from www.ncbi.nlm.nih.gov/pubmed/11743842.

Breitbart, W., Poppito, S., Rosenfeld, B., Vickers, A.J., Li, Y., Abbey, J., . . . Cassileth, B.R. (2012). Pilot randomized controlled trial of individual meaning-centered psychotherapy for patients with advanced cancer. *Journal of Clinical Oncology, 30*(12), 1304–1309. http://doi.org/10.1200/JCO.2011.36.2517.

Breitbart, W., Rosenfeld, B., Gibson, C., Pessin, H., Poppito, S., Nelson, C., . . . Olden, M. (2010). Meaning-centered group psychotherapy for patients with advanced cancer: A pilot randomized controlled trial. *Psycho-Oncology, 19*(1), 21–28. http://doi.org/10.1002/pon.1556.

Breitbart, W., Rosenfeld, B., Pessin, H., Applebaum, A., Kulikowski, J., & Lichtenthal, W.G. (2015). Meaning-centered group psychotherapy: An effective intervention for improving psychological well-being in patients with advanced cancer. *Journal of Clinical Oncology: Official Journal of the American Society of Clinical Oncology, 33*(7), 749–754. http://doi.org/10.1200/JCO.2014.57.2198.

Chibnall, J.T., Bennett, M.L., Videen, S.D., Duckro, P.N., & Miller, D.K. (2004). Identifying barriers to psychosocial spiritual care at the end of life: A physician group study. *American Journal of Hospice & Palliative Care, 21*(6), 419–426.

Chochinov, H.M. (2004). Dignity and psychotherapeutic considerations in end of life care. *Journal of Palliative Care, 20*(3), 134–142.

Chochinov, H.M. (2007). Dignity and the essence of medicine: The A, B, C, and D of dignity conserving care. *BMJ (Clinical Research Ed.), 335*(7612), 184–187. http://doi.org/10.1136/bmj.39244.650926.47.

Chow, E., Tsao, M.N., & Harth, T. (2004). Does psychosocial intervention improve survival in cancer? A meta-analysis. *Palliative Medicine, 18*(1), 25–31. http://doi.org/10.1191/0269216304pm842oa.

Dilworth, S., Higgins, I., Parker, V., Kelly, B., & Turner, J. (2014). Patient and health professional's perceived barriers to the delivery of psychosocial care to adults with cancer: A systematic review. *Psycho-Oncology, 23*(6), 601–612. http://doi.org/10.1002/pon.3474.

Duggleby, W.D., Degner, L., Williams, A., Wright, K., Cooper, D., Popkin, D., & Holtslander, L. (2007). Living with hope: Initial evaluation of a psychosocial hope intervention for older palliative home care patients. *Journal of Pain and Symptom Management, 33*(3), 247–257. http://doi.org/10.1016/j.jpainsymman.2006.09.013.

Frankel, R.M., & Quill, T. (2005). Integrating biopsychosocial and relationship-centered care into mainstream medical practice: A challenge that continues to produce positive results. *Families, Systems, & Health, 23*(4), 413–421. http://doi.org/10.1037/1091-7527.23.4.413.

Garlan, R.W., Butler, L.D., Rosenbaum, E., Siegel, A., & Spiegel, D. (2010). Perceived benefits and psychosocial outcomes of a brief existential family intervention for cancer patients/survivors. *OMEGA—Journal of Death and Dying, 62*(3), 243–268. http://doi.org/10.2190/OM.62.3.c.

Greene, P.B., Philip, E.J., Poppito, S.R., & Schnur, J.B. (2012). Mindfulness and psychosocial care in cancer: Historical context and review of current and potential applications. *Palliative & Supportive Care, 10*(4), 1–8. http://doi.org/10.1017/S1478951511001015.

Greer, J.A., Park, E.R., Prigerson, H.G., & Safren, S.A. (2010). Tailoring Cognitive-Behavioral therapy to treat anxiety comorbid with advanced cancer. *Journal of Cognitive Psychotherapy, 24*(4), 294–313. http://doi.org/10.1891/0889-8391.24.4.294.Tailoring.

Greer, J.A., Traeger, L., Bemis, H., Solis, J., Hendriksen, E.S., Park, E.R., . . . Safren, S. (2012). A pilot randomized controlled trial of brief cognitive-behavioral therapy for anxiety in patients with terminal cancer. *The Oncologist, 17,* 1337–1345.

Guo, Z., Tang, H.-Y., Li, H., Tan, S.-K., Feng, K.-H., Huang, Y.-C., . . . Jiang, W. (2013). The benefits of psychosocial interventions for cancer patients undergoing radiotherapy. *Health and Quality of Life Outcomes, 11*(121), 1–12. http://doi.org/10.1186/1477-7525-11-121.

Holland, J. (2004). An international perspective on the development of psychosocial oncology: Overcoming cultural and attitudinal barriers to improve psychosocial care. *Psycho- Oncology, 13,* 445–459.

Holland, J. (2010). Why psychosocial care is difficult to integrate into routine cancer care: Stigma is the elephant in the room. *Journal of the National Comprehensive Cancer Network, 8*(4), 362–366.

Holland, J., Poppito, S., Nelson, C., Weiss, T., Greenstein, M., Martin, A., . . . Roth, A. (2009). Reappraisal in the eighth life cycle stage: A theoretical psychoeducational intervention in elderly patients with cancer. *Palliative & Supportive Care*, 7(3), 271–279. http://doi.org/10.1017/S1478951509990198.

Howell, D., Mayo, S., Currie, S., Jones, G., Boyle, M., Hack, T., . . . Simpson, J. (2012). Psychosocial health care needs assessment of adult cancer patients: A consensus-based guideline. *Supportive Care in Cancer*, 20(12), 3343–3354. http://doi.org/10.1007/s00520-012-1468-x.

Hudson, P. L., Remedios, C., & Thomas, K. (2010). A systematic review of psychosocial interventions for family carers of palliative care patients. *BMC Palliative Care*, 9, 17. http://doi.org/10.1186/1472-684X-9-17.

Institute of Medicine (2007). *Cancer care for the whole patient: Meeting psychosocial health needs*. Washington, D.C.: National Academy Press.

Jacobsen, P. B. (2009). Promoting evidence-based psychosocial care for cancer patients. *Psycho-Oncology*, 18(1), 6–13. http://doi.org/10.1002/pon.1468.

Jacobsen, P. B., Holland, J., & Steensma, D. P. (2012). Caring for the whole patient: The science of psychosocial care. *Journal of Clinical Oncology*, 30(11), 1151–1153.

Kissane, D. W., Bloch, S., Smith, G. C., Miach, P., Clarke, D. M., Ikin, J., . . . McKenzie, D. (2003). Cognitive-existential group psychotherapy for women with primary breast cancer: A randomised controlled trial. *Psycho-Oncology*, 12(6), 532–546. http://doi.org/10.1002/pon.683.

Kissane, D. W., Grabsch, B., Clarke, D. M., Christie, G., Clifton, D., Gold, S., . . . Smith, G. C. (2004). Supportive-expressive group therapy: The transformation of existential ambivalence into creative living while enhancing adherence to anti-cancer therapies. *Psycho-Oncology*, 13(11), 755–768. http://doi.org/10.1002/pon.798.

Kissane, D. W., Grabsch, B., Clarke, D. M., Smith, G. C., Love, A. W., Bloch, S., . . . Li, Y. (2007). Supportive-expressive group therapy for women with metastatic breast cancer: Survival and psychosocial outcome from a randomized controlled trial. *Psycho-Oncology*, 16(4), 277–286. http://doi.org/10.1002/pon.

Lee, V. (2008). The existential plight of cancer: Meaning making as a concrete approach to the intangible search for meaning. *Support Care Cancer*, 16(7), 779–785. http://doi.org/10.1007/s00520-007-0396-7.

Lee, V., Cohen, S. R., Edgar, L., Laizner, A. M., & Gagnon, A. J. (2006). Meaning-making and psychological adjustment to cancer: Development of an intervention and pilot results. *Oncology Nursing Forum*, 33(2), 291–302. http://doi.org/10.1188/06.ONF.291-302.

Miller, D. K., Chibnall, J. T., Videen, S. D., & Duckro, P. N. (2005). Supportive-affective group experience for persons with life-threatening illness: Reducing spiritual, psychological, and death-related distress in dying patients. *Journal of Palliative Medicine*, 8(2), 333–343. http://doi.org/10.1089/jpm.2005.8.333.

Nissim, R., Freeman, E., Lo, C., Zimmermann, C., Gagliese, L., Rydall, A., . . . Rodin, G. (2012). Managing cancer and living meaningfully (CALM): A qualitative study of a brief individual psychotherapy for individuals with advanced cancer. *Palliative Medicine*, 26(5), 713–721. http://doi.org/10.1177/0269216311425096.

Richardson, P. (2014). Spirituality, religion and palliative care. *Annals of Palliative Medicine*, 3(3), 150–159. http://doi.org/10.3978/j.issn.2224-5820.2014.07.05.

Rodin, G. (2013). Research on psychological and social factors in palliative care: An invited commentary. *Palliative Medicine*, 27(10), 925–931. http://doi.org/10.1177/0269216313499961.

Steinhauser, K. E., Alexander, S. C., Byock, I. R., George, L. K., Olsen, M. K., & Tulsky, J. A. (2008). Do preparation and life completion discussions improve functioning and quality of life in seriously ill patients? Pilot randomized control trial. *Journal of Palliative Medicine*, 11(9), 1234–1240. http://doi.org/10.1089/jpm.2008.0078.

Steinhauser, K. E., Christakis, N. A., Clipp, E. C., McNeilly, M., McIntyre, L., & Tulsky, J. A. (2000). Factors considered important at the end of life by patients, family, physicians, and other care providers. *JAMA: The Journal of the American Medical Association, 284*(19), 2476–2482. http://doi.org/10.1001/jama.284.19.2476.

Weisman, A. D. (1974). *The realization of death*. New York & London: Jason Aronson Inc.

Werth Jr., J. L., Gordon, J. R., & Johnson Jr., R. J. (2002). Psychosocial issues near the end of life. *Aging & Mental Health, 6*(4), 402–412. http://doi.org/10.1080/1 360786021000007027.

6 Spirituality, Religion, and the Good Death

> Spirituality concerns a person's relationship with *transcendence*. Therefore, genuinely holistic health care must address the totality of the patient's relational existence—physical, psychological, social, and spiritual.
>
> (Sulmasy, 2002, p. 24)

6.1 DEFINING SPIRITUALITY AND RELIGION

> Being spiritual has become a way of putting distance between one's self and religion, while holding onto something regarded as good. Thus spirituality is defined against what it is not. Inevitably this means that what is seen as the negative about religion will be influential in what is seen as spiritual.
>
> (King & Koenig, 2009, p. 17)

A clear distinction between religion and spirituality has been amply and variously discussed in the literature. A large, growing literature explores spirituality and religion in the healthcare context, particularly as it concerns the practice of oncology. The definitions of religion and of spirituality have been a subject of much debate and some consensus, globally influenced by culture and demography. Until approximately the 1990s, religion was the umbrella term to encompass both concepts (Peterman et al., 2002; Peterman et al., 2014). Recent clinical research has widely tested the related concepts of meaning, peace, faith, purpose, and hope in relation to religion and spirituality, in an attempt to characterize their definitions and usage. One realizes that, reading a piece on religion written in the 1990s or earlier on the topic of religion and healthcare, use of the term religion in that early instance might in fact include spirituality.

The roots of the word "religion" come from the Latin *religare*, which means "to bind together". The concept of religion organizes the collective spiritual experiences of a group of people into a system of beliefs and practices. Religious involvement, or religiosity, refers to the degree of participation in, or adherence to, the beliefs and practices of an organized religion

(Surbone & Baider, 2010). Religion provides "a set of beliefs, practices, and language that characterizes a community that is searching for transcendent meaning in a particular way, generally on the basis of belief in a deity" (Sulmasy, 2002, p. 25). Religions grant people a way to find meaning and hope, social support and guidance, a context in which to understand our personal suffering within the greater picture of human experience, and a supportive community to help individuals cope with the complexities of life, particularly illness, loss, death, and dying. Religion offers people values, rituals, and concepts that assist people in connecting to one another as part of a healing process during a time of suffering (Puchalski & O'Donnell, 2005). In contrast, spirituality is a broader, more personal concept than that of religion.

Kearney and Mount (2000) likened spirituality to a "dimension of personhood, a part of our being while religion was seen as a construct of human making that . . . enables conceptualization and expression of spirituality" (p. 359). Personhood defines the essence of humanity (Kaut, 2002).

As an exercise in clarity, Figure 6.1 highlights the predominant definitions of religion and spirituality found in a relatively comprehensive review of the healthcare literature, in order briefly to compare and contrast the definitions found. In brief, spirituality is defined as a universal human characteristic, a way to find meaning and purpose in life, to experience connection to one's self, others, or the sacred. Religion is seen as an expression of spirituality, a set of organized beliefs that is shared within a community (Puchalski, 2012). Terminally ill patients may utilize their spiritual or religious beliefs and values as a way to understand their illness; find meaning in the midst of their suffering; find hope in their grief, loss, and distress; and find inner peace.

SPIRITUALITY	RELIGION
Spiritus: breath, the animating life force (Bryson, 2004)	*Religare*: to bind together
A personal search for existential meaning allowing one to make sense of a situation (Best et al., 2014); a personal search for meaning and purpose in life (Peterman et al., 2002)	Beliefs/practices that facilitate making meaning. A formal expression of spirituality (Best et al., 2014)
Spirituality describes "the depths of human life", the part that seeks healing; a search for significance/meaning not dependent on a theology; a broad personal concept, a sense of connectedness to a personal God (Chochinov & McCann, 2005, S105-7).	A set of organized beliefs about God; an organized faith system, beliefs, worship, religious rituals and relationship with a divine being (in Sinclair et al., 2012)
Frankl & meaning/transcendence (1984): 1) give to the world (creation); 2) take from the world by experiences and encounters; 3) how one faces predicaments of fate.	
A conscious process of self-reflection that allows the experience of transcendent meaning and person values (Valchon et al., 2009)	Religion as "codified, institutionalized and relatively narrow expression of spirituality (Walter, 2002).
Connection with the transcendent dimension of existence (Peterman et al., 2002); concerns a person's relationship with the transcendent (Sulmasy, 2002)	A system of beliefs or spiritual experiences characterizing a community, based on belief in a deity.
King & Koenig (2009): 4 components of definition of spirituality: 1) Belief: conviction about existence that goes beyond the material world; 2) Practice: occurs without conscious awareness of the spiritual realm addressed; 3) Awareness: of being moved intellectually and/or emotionally; 4) Experience: may include diffusion of the mind, loss of ego boundaries and a change in orientation from self towards or beyond the material world.	Religiosity: the degree of participation in or adherence to the beliefs and practices of an organized religion
Puchalski (2000): that which allows a person to experience transcendent meaning in life. (2012): Has to do with arts, humanism, cultural beliefs and practices; the inner life of a person; a way to find meaning and purpose; how to experience connectedness to self, others, sacred or significant; relationship with transcendent; a universal human characteristic; source of strength in dealing with illness. Helps people find hope in the midst of despair (2000)	Offers believers values, rituals and concepts that help them connect to one another; offers spiritual ways of understanding suffering (Puchalski, 2012) One's faith community (Cohen & Koenig, 2003)
A dimension of personhood, "a part of our being" (Kearney & Mount, 2000)	"a construct of human making" that enables expression of spirituality (Kearney & Mount, 2000).

"Overlapping, interconnected constructions experienced by whole persons" (Chochinov & McCann, 2005, p. S106)

Figure 6.1 Definitions of Spirituality/Religion (Author)

In 2009, a consensus conference on the topic of improving the quality of spiritual care as a dimension of palliative care agreed on a definition of spirituality as: "the aspect of humanity that refers to the ways individuals seek and express meaning as well as the way they experience their connectedness to the moment, to self, to others, to nature, and to the significant or sacred" (Puchalski et al., 2009, p. 887). Recommendations were set forth that specified the spiritual care models that may be used by clinical sites.

Indeed, Chochinov and Cann (2005) observed that increased secularism has seen a lessening of the explicit and implicit religious connotations associated with the term "spirituality". Spirituality has aligned itself with a sense of connectedness to a personal God and a search for significance and meaning that does not necessarily depend upon a specific theology. The genesis of such significance will vary from person to person, but what religion and spirituality hold in common is their "ability to imbue life with an overarching sense of purpose and meaning, including a sustained investment in life itself" (Chochinov & Cann, 2005, p. S107).

The interest in attending to the religious/spiritual needs of dying persons is a relatively recent phenomenon among healthcare practitioners globally. In the United States, the SUPPORT study (SUPPORT Principal Investigators, 1995) revealed the inadequacy of the management of pain and suffering inherent in end-of-life care, and much of the suffering patients experience is spiritual suffering (Puchalski, 2002, 2012). Steinhauser et al.'s study that investigated the wants/needs of clinicians, patients, and caregivers, "In Search of a Good Death", found that control of pain and attention to spiritual issues ranked first in importance with patients, nurses, social workers, and chaplains, but that spiritual issues ranked third in importance with physicians (Steinhauser, Christakis et al., 2000; Steinhauser, Clipp et al., 2000). Hospice has always led the way in placing a great importance on issues of spirituality, while palliative medicine strives to care for the whole patient and for their family, including issues of spirituality.

The consideration of a patient's spiritual values is seen as being critical to achieving a good death. Good palliative care concerns not only the relief of pain and physical symptoms, but must also be extended to include psychiatric, psychosocial, existential, and spiritual domains of end-of-life care. Puchalski (2000) defined spirituality as "that which allows a person to experience transcendent meaning in life. . . . Whatever beliefs and values give a person a sense of meaning and purpose in life" (p. 129).

Dying patients need to be reassured that they have value by virtue of being human, at a time when their reduced productivity, dependence, and altered appearance have called into question their ultimate value as persons and may even have caused them to doubt their own intrinsic value (Sulmasy, 2006, p. 1387). Regardless of religious affiliation, the need of the dying to know that they are valued is a powerful spiritual need. Despite a patient's spiritual bent, for the patient, dying raises the questions of the value and meaning of his or her life, suffering, and death:

> Questions of value are often subsumed under the term, dignity. Questions of meaning are often subsumed under the word "hope". Questions of relationship are often expressed in the need for "forgiveness". To die believing that one's life and death have been of no value is the ultimate indignity. For the physician to ignore these questions is to abandon the patient at the individual's greatest hour of need.
>
> (Sulmasy, 2002, p. 26)

Sulmasy, an early proponent of the need to include spirituality in healthcare, reiterated the distinction, made by many scholars, between religion and spirituality: spirituality refers to an individual's or a group's relationship with the transcendent, however that may be construed. Spirituality is about the search for transcendent meaning (Sulmasy, 2002, p. 25). Many people express their spirituality in religious practice, whereas others express spirituality through their relationship with nature, art, music, or a set of philosophical beliefs that they may share with friends and family.

In an attempt to define spirituality, a search of the literature of the last ten years yielded a conceptual analysis of spirituality at the end of life (Vachon et al., 2009). The analysis yielded 11 dimensions of the concept of end-of-life spirituality, namely: (1) meaning and purpose in life; (2) self-transcendence; (3) transcendence with a higher being; (4) feelings of communion and mutuality; (5) beliefs and faith; (6) hope; (7) attitude toward death; (8) appreciation of life; (9) reflection upon fundamental values; (10) the developmental nature of spirituality; and (11) its conscious aspect. Vachon et al. (2009) therefore suggested that spirituality be described as a dynamic process that evolves in time and is often triggered, especially in the context of serious illness, by confrontation with either death itself or illness, which then challenges one's belief system. Vachon et al. proposed that the "consciousness of the *transcending* dimensions, the capacity to recognize the singularity of specific moments and the capacity to reflect upon values and priorities are what makes an experience spiritual" (p. 56). In conclusion, the authors defined spirituality as a developmental and conscious process, characterized by two movements of transcendence; either deep within the self or beyond the self (p. 56).

Steinhauser et al. (2006) conducted an evidence-based study whose purpose was to explore the construct of being at peace, which offered clinicians a means of assessing patients' spirituality. The results of the study revealed that resolution amongst the psychosocial, biomedical, and spiritual domains of patient experience often preceded the patient's subjective experience of peacefulness. Thus, asking if a patient or family member is at peace offers a straightforward way for a clinician to explore spiritual issues within the limited time of end-of-life care. The clinician then is able to direct patients/ families to specialized care, such as chaplaincy, while understanding the types of distress their patient is struggling with, such as life completion. This type of intervention can result in the interdisciplinary scope of psychosocial care, as well as affording communications between clinicians and patients.

6.2 ELEMENTS OF SPIRITUALITY: TRANSCENDENCE, MEANING, AND GOOD DEATH

> Human existence is not authentic unless it is lived in terms of self-*transcendence* . . . self-*transcendence* is the essence of existence.
>
> (Frankl, 1966, p. 104)

Receiving a diagnosis of a terminal illness changes peoples' lives forever, raising issues of spirituality and of existential concerns, triggering questions of meaning, purpose, and hope. Spirituality is recognized by healthcare accrediting agencies as an essential aspect of quality of life, along with physical, emotional, and psychosocial well-being (The Health and Human Services Guidelines for Spiritual and Religious Care, the Clinical Standards for Specialist Palliative Care, National Institutes for Clinical Excellence (NICE) Guidelines, and the revised World Health Organization [WHO] definition of palliative care; see also Puchalski et al., 2006). Spirituality can facilitate self-transcendence, enabling an aging person to grow in face of terminal diagnoses, loss, disability, and dying (Byock, 1996; Ardelt et al., 2013). Chibnall et al. (2002) have shown spirituality to be related to greater physical, psychological, and relational health.

All people seek meaning and purpose in life, and this search is intensified when someone faces serious illness and death. In noting the abundant definitions separating the realms of religion and of spirituality, Walter (1997) identified spirituality as the search for meaning (p. 22). This concept of spirituality is founded in the idea that human beings have a desire to transcend hardship and suffering, particularly at the end of life. Transcendence may be achieved by "searching for and/or in one's inherited or chosen religious beliefs and ideas" (Kellehear, 2000, p. 150). Thus, many scholars express that the common feature of spirituality or spiritual care is the sense of transcendence, a way to live one's life at a deeper level. Spirituality may be understood as "a person's search for ultimate meaning in the context of religious values, beliefs and practices or other expressions such as relationships with families, communities or work, as well as the arts, nature and the humanities" (Association of American Medical Colleges Contemporary Issues in Medicine: Communication in Medicine, 1999, p. 27, in Puchalski et al., 2006, p. 398).

Vachon et al. (2009) defined spirituality in terms of self-*transcendence*, involving profound self-reflection and the will to live according to one's personal values. Self-*transcendence* thereby allows one to give meaning to events as well as to discover a unique purpose and global meaning to life and to death.

Frankl believed in three principal ways a person may find meaning: by giving to the world in terms of creations; by taking from the world in terms of encounters and experiences with others; and "in the stance taken toward a predicament the fate of which cannot be changed" (in Coward & Reed, 1996, p. 280), in this case, that of terminal illness and impending death. Such aspects are part of the quality of self-transcendence that may help to promote healing at the end of life and contribute to a good death.

Coward and Reed (1996) provided results of studies demonstrating clinical and empirical evidence for the efficacy of self-*transcendence* in healing elderly people facing aging, chronic disease, or terminal illness. Initially, Reed studied spiritual perspectives of self-*transcendence* and found them to be strongly and positively related to subjective well-being of terminal patients (Davison & Jhangri, 2013). Psychosocial forms of self-*transcendence*, such as healing insights about life and death, correlated and predicted healing, including relief of depression and suicidal ideation. Body *transcendence*, the ability to transcend the physical ailments and limitations of aging, was also found to be significant. These elements of transcendence, then, facilitate a search for meaning at the end of life, smoothing the way for a good death.

Sulmasy (2002) proposed the possibility for healing in a dying person by experiencing love, being seen as valuable even though not economically productive, and by accepting the role of teacher while providing valuable life lessons to survivors. The ability to grapple with the *transcendent* idea of each of these questions about existence, meaning, value, and relationship also presents dying people an opportunity for healing. Individuals struggling with end-of-life issues must expend considerable energy to attain self-*transcendence*, but such efforts have provided healing and potentially initiated a start towards a good death.

McGrath's studies of Australian hospice patients (2003a & 2003b), which aimed to clarify an understanding of how individuals respond spiritually to the effect of serious illness, affirmed a dichotomy between religion and spirituality. Patients did not bring with them a sense of preformed religious ideas of their serious illnesses; instead they developed a sense of their own spiritual views from life experience to deal with it.

6.3 RELIGIOUS COPING/SPIRITUAL WELL-BEING, QUALITY OF LIFE, AND THE GOOD DEATH

> Spiritual well-being is a determinant of whole health and, by extension, quality of life.
>
> (Puchalski, 2012, p. iii51).

The SUPPORT study and evidence of other countries' suboptimal care of terminally ill patients led, in the 1990s, to the establishment of clinical care pathways and identifying other means of improving patients' quality of life with clinical research. Since then, recognition has grown regarding the importance of identifying what matters to the quality of life (QOL) of patients with life-threatening disease. Such patients must cope with the full range of physical and psychological symptoms of their illness on their family members. Consequently, the strategies that patients use to cope with these challenges are an important influence on how they manage their lives, and, ultimately, the quality of their deaths.

Quality of life research has passed its infancy and the established domains of physical, social/family, emotional, and functional status are the well-established core characteristics of QOL assessments. Now, momentum is gaining for adoption of the biopsychosocial-spiritual model of QOL assessment. Individuals living with terminal illness face considerable challenges that can significantly hamper their quality of life. Religion and spirituality have become increasingly important as patients approach the end of life and these concepts are well-recognized as factors that affect patients QOL, quality of care, and satisfaction with palliative care (Astrow et al., 2007; M. Balboni et al., 2013; T. Balboni et al., 2007; Davison & Jhangri, 2013; Puchalski & Romer, 2000; Winkelman et al., 2011). To that end, research has shown that religion and spirituality have come to play a large part in improving coping and QOL in advanced disease (T. Balboni et al., 2007; Tarakeshwar et al., 2006; Brady et al., 1999; McClain et al., 2003; Nelson et al., 2002).

In an early lecture at Baylor University Medical Center, Puchalski (2001) discussed the impact of spirituality on healthcare. She maintained that spirituality is essential in the measuring of quality of life scores: "Positive reports on those measures—a meaningful personal existence, fulfillment of life goals and a feeling that life . . . had been worthwhile—correlated with a good quality of life" (p. 353) in patients with advanced disease. Quality of life consists of multiple facets, including how an individual is faring spiritually, not merely one's physical, psychological, and interpersonal states (Efficace & Marrone, 2002). Spiritual well-being enables severely ill people to enjoy life even in the face of a considerable symptom load. A large trial (Brady et al., 1999) featuring a diverse population of people with cancer and HIV found spiritual well-being to be related to the ability to enjoy life even in the midst of symptoms. Results of a study investigating associations between spiritual well-being and depression in patients with advanced cancer indicate that spiritual well-being may be an asset to cancer survivors and may function as a buffer against maladaptive coping and stress (Ando et al., 2008; Gonzalez et al., 2014). Such study results support the move to the biopsychosocial-spiritual model for QOL in end-of-life care.

When the goals of care change from biomedical/curative to psychosocial/comfort, improving or maintaining quality of life becomes crucial. Patients have identified multiple domains of QOL indicators, including the quality of their palliative care, relationships with family and friends, engagement in activities and hobbies, general outlook on life, and consideration of future issues related to their death (Steinhauser et al., 2000; Vig & Pearlman, 2003). Patients with terminal or life-threatening illness struggle with coping, physically and emotionally, but also with the spiritual and existential issues of their illness (Delgado-Guay, 2014). The incorporation of aspects of spirituality or of religion in palliative care treatment have been shown to help with a patient's emotional coping when facing life-limiting illness (Best et al., 2014; Daaleman & VandeCreek, 2000; Efficace & Marrone, 2002; Kearney & Mount 2000; McGrath, 2003a, 2003b; Puchalski, 2002; Puchalski & O'Donnell, 2005; Walter, 1997). A strong doctor–patient relationship likewise contributes to emotional coping (Best et al., 2014).

Whereas spirituality may be viewed as a way to identify meaning and the sacred, religion is a construct of human making that enables the conceptualization and expression of spirituality. Religious coping has been found to play an important role in the quality of life of patients with cancer (Tarakeshwar et al., 2006; Phelps et al., 2009). Within the framework of spirituality and religion, religious coping is found to be a distinct entity, providing prayer, meditation, and religious study as meaningful and comforting factors in coping with advanced illness (Phelps et al., 2009; Richardson, 2014). Positive religious coping refers to the way in which patients use their religious beliefs to understand and adapt to life stressors, to make sense of and find meaning in their illness (Richardson, 2014, p. 154). Studies have found that religion and spirituality generally play a positive role in patients coping with illnesses such as cancer or HIV (Breitbart & Rosenfeld, 1999; Nelson et al., 2002). Park and Folkman (1997) described meaning as a "general life orientation, as personal significance, as causality, as a coping mechanism, and as an outcome" (in Breitbart, 2001, p. 4).

A study (Lin & Bauer-Wu, 2003) on psychospiritual well-being among individuals with advanced cancer revealed six essential topics through which religion/spirituality influenced well-being: self-awareness, coping and adjusting effectively with stress, relationships and connectedness with others, sense of faith, sense of empowerment, confidence, and living with meaning and hope. Patients with an enhanced sense of psychospiritual well-being are able to cope more effectively with the process of terminal illness and to find meaning in the experience.

Positive religious coping was found to be associated with better quality of life and improvements in health, while negative religious coping was found to be associated with worse QOL (Tarakeshwar et al., 2006; Peteet & M. Balboni, 2013). However, a 2007 study found that while spiritual support is associated with better QOL, many advanced cancer patients' spiritual needs are not supported by religious communities or by the medical system, and religious individuals more frequently want aggressive measures used to extend life. Prognostic awareness, family and social support, autonomy, hope, and meaning in life all contribute to positive psychospiritual well-being and to the possibility of achieving a good death (T. Balboni et al., 2007; Tarakeshwar et al., 2006).

Spiritual beliefs help patients to cope with their disease and to face death, and are associated with better quality of life (T. Balboni et al., 2007; Delgado-Guay et al., 2011; Peteet & M. Balboni, 2013) and lower levels of depression (Nelson et al., 2002; Gonzalez et al., 2014). Spiritual commitment is apt to help patients recover from illness and surgery, because people who worry less have better health outcomes, and spirituality may assist those who worry less (Puchalski & Romer, 2000; Puchalski, 2001). Puchalski urged physicians to deliver compassionate care by focusing on patients' physical, emotional, and spiritual suffering. Healthcare professionals should try to engage patients on a spiritual level if they are in the midst of despair. As the physical and technological aspects of modern day healthcare take precedence over more holistic needs, spirituality may become an important intervention in supportive comfort care after "there is nothing more we can do" is pronounced (Puchalski et al., 2006, p. 399). Looking to a belief system, another person, or activity can help patients transcend physical pain and change the focus of their lives to something outside their physical suffering. Thus, all healthcare professionals have the obligation to communicate with each patient in their care about his or her spiritual needs and concerns. If a patient is in spiritual distress, their healthcare can be compromised (Peteet & M. Balboni, 2013). Addressing all four dimensions of care—physical, emotional, social, and spiritual—is necessary to ensure the best end-of-life medical care.

The Religion and Spirituality in Cancer Care study demonstrated that spiritual concerns are common in the setting of advanced cancer. Spirituality and religion have become a focus of palliative care and mental health research to identify the reasons that some terminally ill patients become depressed during the terminal stage of illness. The relationship of spiritual concerns to quality of life in patients with advanced cancer has been found to be associated with poorer QOL among advanced cancer patients (Winkelman et al., 2011). Patients experiencing spiritual concerns, whether spiritual struggles (e.g., feeling abandoned by God) or spiritual seeking (e.g., thinking about what gives meaning to life) experience poorer psychological QOL (p. 1026). Nevertheless, spiritual pain, a concept with many definitions and attributed meanings, was significantly associated with a lower self-rated religiosity and a trend toward lower self-rated spirituality (Delgado-Guay et al., 2011).

Symptomatic relief of a patient's pain—physical or spiritual—at the end of life, as well as facilitating that patient's reconciliation with family and friends, represents genuine healing within the biopsychosocial-spiritual model. Each person must live and die according to the answer each gives to the question of whether life or death has a meaning that transcends both life and death (Sulmasy, 2002, p. 26). The act of healing is the facilitation of the dying person's struggle with this question. The very important instrument, the McGill Quality of Life questionnaire (MQOL), supports these researchers' hypothesis (Cohen et al., 1996) that the existential domain plays an important part of an individual's quality of life.

Cohen et al.'s 2001 study demonstrated the importance to terminally ill patients in palliative care units of themes relating to spirituality, existential well-being, and religious beliefs. These themes were the perception that quality of life had been improved through enhanced spiritual awareness; an increase in awareness of thoughts about the afterlife; an increase in the sense of hope; growing acceptance; and changes in involvement in religious rituals (Cohen et al., 2001, p. 368). Patients also became less anxious and depressed, and experienced an increase in existential/spiritual well-being.

Clinicians are charged with discerning and implementing their patients' spiritual concerns in goals of treatment for end-of-life (EOL) care (Lo et al., 2002). Studies indicate that patients want their physicians to be attentive to religious/spiritual needs (Sulmasy, 2002; Vallurupalli et al., 2012), and that spiritual support from medical providers is associated with improved quality of life (T. Balboni et al., 2007), satisfaction with medical care (Astrow et al., 2007), and lower rates of aggressive EOL care (T. Balboni et al., 2010). Should physicians ignore the spiritual concerns of their patients, clinicians are "asking many patients to alienate themselves from beliefs that deeply define them, at times of great vulnerability, as the price for receiving attention for their physical needs" (Sulmasy, 2006, p. 1388; Sharma et al., 2012). Often, however, clinicians are hesitant to inquire about their patients' spiritual and religious beliefs, possibly due to their "own spiritual and existential struggles, not just with the idea of death, but also with the ultimate impotence of medicine as a cure for death" (Sulmasy, 2006, p. 1388). Other physicians hesitate to elicit this information because they fear they lack the time or capability to do so. The question of who ought to facilitate a patient's spiritual healing is unclear; nevertheless, patients have expressed a desire for their physicians to be involved (Sulmasy, 2002; Post et al., 2000). Moadel et al. (1999) conducted a study regarding patients' attitudes to the spiritual dimensions of care. Patients in this study identified the nature, prevalence, and correlates of spiritual and existential needs among an ethnically-diverse, urban sample of cancer patients ($n = 248$) ". . . [who] indicated wanting help with: overcoming my fears (51%), finding hope (42%), finding meaning in life (40%), finding spiritual resources (39%); or someone to talk to about: finding peace of mind (43%), the meaning of life (28%), and dying and death (25%)" (p. 378).

Efforts are under way to establish interventions to positively impact the spiritual well-being and quality of life of patients with advanced cancer. Piderman et al. (2014) conducted a randomized controlled trial of patients with advanced cancer receiving radiation therapy. The results indicated that the multidisciplinary intervention, which included a spiritual component, can maintain the spiritual QOL of patients with advanced cancer during radiation therapy. The study supports a growing literature on structured interventions augmented with spiritual components that found interventions to be effective in positively impacting the spiritual well-being and QOL of patients with advanced and metastatic cancer (Piderman et al., 2015).

Another such intervention, meaning-centered group psychotherapy (MCGP), was tested by Breitbart et al. (2015). The study sought to investigate whether psychological distress was reduced and spiritual well-being improved in patients with advanced or terminal cancer. The need to cope with advanced cancer often causes serious psychological distress in many patients. Psychological distress is marked by depression and hopelessness, as well as a loss of spiritual well-being, existential distress, and even a desire for hastened death. Therefore, the need to assess and treat psychological disorders is a crucial component of care in oncology and palliative care settings. The results of this randomized controlled study provided strong evidence that MCGP is an effective intervention in improving quality of life and spiritual well-being, and reducing depression, hopelessness, and desire for hastened death in individuals with advanced stage cancer. The MCGP intervention appears to be effective in targeting critical elements of existential, spiritual, and psychological distress in patients with advanced cancer. Patients confronting a terminal illness often experience these strong feelings of distress, so an empirically supported intervention such as MCGP proved to be an important tool for use by clinicians who struggle to help their patients with such difficult challenges (Breitbart et al., 2015, pp. 753–4).

The principle of patient autonomy mandates that physicians respect the decisions of competent patients, which are often based on religious and spiritual beliefs. Cancer patients reporting that their spiritual needs are not well supported by their healthcare team have higher end-of-life (EOL) costs, particularly among minorities and high religious coping patients (T. Balboni et al., 2010; T. Balboni et al., 2011). A recent study investigated whether spiritual support from religious communities influences the medical care of terminally ill patients at the end of life (T. Balboni et al., 2013). The results report that terminally ill patients who received strong support from religious communities were less likely to use hospice care, more likely to receive aggressive measures at the end of life, and to die in an ICU. Conversely, among the patients who received support from their religious communities but also received spiritual support from medical teams, higher use of hospice, fewer aggressive interventions, and fewer ICU deaths were found. Also, end-of-life discussions were associated with fewer aggressive patient interventions. Clearly, these data reveal a mandate for the inclusion of spiritual care in end-of-life medical care guidelines, and can also contribute to patient's good death.

6.4 THE SPIRITUAL HISTORY

What physicians might do is to take a spiritual history, a way to elicit a patient's spiritual and religious beliefs and concerns; to try to understand them; to relate the patient's beliefs to decisions that need to be made regarding care; to attempt to reach some preliminary conclusions about whether the patient's religious coping is positive or negative; and to refer to pastoral care or the patient's own clergy as seems appropriate (Sulmasy, 2006, p. 1388). Sulmasy (2006) and Puchalski and Romer (2000) each advocated the incorporation of a spiritual assessment into standard medical history-taking. Its use is valuable to a patient–physician relationship by opening the door to conversations about spirituality and religion important to the patient. A spiritual history only provides a backdrop against which a clinician may understand the pressing spiritual questions that dying patients face (Sulmasy, 2006, p. 1389). The presence of unmet spiritual needs was found to correlate with lower satisfaction of care and with a lower satisfaction with quality of care (Astrow et al., 2007; Peteet & M. Balboni, 2013).

Puchalski and Romer see the spiritual history as a means of returning medicine to the "compassionate, caregiving roots of the patient-doctor relationship" (2000, p. 129; Puchalski & O'Donnell, 2005) and helping providers understand whatever role spirituality plays in the patient–doctor relationship itself. A spiritual history assesses a patient's religious or spiritual background and is typically done as part of an initial clinical evaluation. Spiritual histories empower physicians and nurses to advocate for the religious/spiritual needs of their patients, such as through chaplaincy referrals, support groups, and more careful navigation of the intersection between religion/spirituality and medical decisions, especially in the context of end-of-life care (Epstein-Peterson et al., 2014).

The Spiritual Assessment tool developed by Puchalski and Romer is known as FICA, an acronym that can be used to remember what the clinician may ask (2000, pp. 130–2):

F represents faith or beliefs of the patient, either religion or spirituality
I stands for the importance or influence of the faith or beliefs of the patient
C refers to community, whether religious or spiritual
A implies the thought of how to address the previous information

Findings (Borneman et al., 2010) suggest that the FICA tool is a feasible one for clinical assessment of spirituality, as most patients rated faith or belief as very important in their lives. The FICA tool is patient-centered, guided by the extent to which patients wish to disclose/discuss their personal sense of spirituality. FICA quantitative ratings and qualitative comments were closely correlated with items from the quality of life tools assessing aspects of spirituality. These ratings show that addressing spiritual needs and concerns in clinical settings is critical in enhancing quality of life at the end of life, especially in the context of terminal illness, and ought to become a routine part of clinical care (T. Balboni et al., 2007). Doing so can add to the potential of achieving a good death.

However, while the latest information from clinical trials in the Boston area (Epstein-Peterson et al., 2014) reinforced the long-standing importance to terminal patients of participation by their physicians in religious/spiritual support, findings revealed "low frequencies of all types of SC [spiritual care] as reported by patients with incurable cancer and their nurse/physician care providers. . . . When provided, the most common SC type reported was encouraging R/S [religious/spiritual] beliefs" (p. 6). The core elements of spiritual care, spiritual histories and chaplaincy referrals, together only comprised 26 percent of SC provided. Clinicians only infrequently provide spiritual care to patients with advanced cancer and few referrals to chaplaincy, in spite of evidence demonstrating its importance to patients, as reported in this study. One might question the influence of demographics on these findings, of how representative these findings from an urban population within a group of sophisticated medical centers are, and therefore their significance as representative of religious/spiritual palliative care at this point in time in the United States.

Another compelling means of contributing to the spiritual needs of patients at the end of life summed up many of the findings and improvements found in quality of life research since the 1990s, representing another possible intervention for religious/spiritual care. In a 2012 qualitative study (Sinclair et al.), Canadian palliative care professionals identified spiritual care as both a specialized care domain and as a philosophy of care that informs and is embedded within physical and psychosocial care of patients at the end of life. The study establishes the central role of clinician presence in interactions with patients across all care domains in end of life care, as well as four other bedside skills that are core to the provision of spiritual care: listening, sight, touch, and speech. Clinician presence with patients is described as:

> The fifth bedside skill, presence, was the foundation upon which the other four categories were grounded. Presence was seen as the outward radiance of an individual's essence or soul. Presence was not based on technical competence, spiritual awareness or self-assessed spirituality, but the expression of clinicians' character, beliefs, behaviour and giftedness within their clinical practice. Participants believed that presence was an innate aspect of humanity, experienced relationally in terms of being with rather than doing for.
>
> (Sinclair et al., 2012, p. 323)

Sinclair et al. took a cue from Saunders's (2001) expressions "being with" rather than "doing for" in mandating ways to care for the spiritual needs of dying patients. While so saying is nearly obvious in its truth and realness, an eventual good death within such circumstances can almost be pictured.

Integrating spiritual assessment and basic communication in end-of-life care may occur at different levels, ranging from asking patients to respond to basic questions about their spiritual beliefs and needs, to engaging at a personal level with patients who try to involve their clinicians in the spiritual dimension of their care, to intervening as part of a spiritual team, the implementation of which can help achieve a good death.

6.5 SPIRITUAL COPING AND HOPE

> Those who know how close the connection is between the state of mind of a man—his courage and hope or lack of them—and the state of immunity of his body will understand that the sudden loss of hope and courage can have a deadly effect.
>
> (Frankl, 1984, pp. 96–7)

Dufault and Martocchio have defined hope as a multidimensional dynamic life force characterized by a confident yet uncertain expectation of achieving a future good (Dufault & Martocchio, 1985, p. 380, as cited in Alidina & Tettero, 2010), which, to the hoping person, is realistically possible and personally significant (Duggleby et al., 2013). In Weisman's (1972) view, having hope means that we have confidence in the *desirability* of surviving (p. 20). An important coping strategy, hope enables an individual to adapt to a difficult situation that allows personal adjustments during suffering. Sherwin Nuland (1994) defined hope as the "expectation of a good that is yet to be, a perception of a future condition in which a desired goal will be achieved" (p. 223).

At the onset, one hopes for cure or restoration of health (Eliott & Olver, 2009), but in terminal illness, when the possibility of a cure is gone, hope resides in the skill of physicians to alter the course of disease and to prolong life. At life's end, hope endures even though science can do no more; however, the focus of hope is redefined and becomes the hope of finding meaning in life, as it was lived, as well as in the time that remains (Hawthorne & Yurkovich, 2004).

Spirituality helps people find hope in the midst of their suffering. Hope enables terminally ill patients to face their uncertain future and adapt to their mortality. Hope eases the ability to endure suffering, giving life meaning, direction, and a degree of optimism. Hope nourishes people with psychological and physical difficulties to set goals and priorities, reestablish spirituality, and to continue to live. Hope facilitates *transcendence* in order to establish new meaning and purpose to life. The concept of hope is common to each of us and unique for each of us, but is complex to define. However, using the technique of concept analysis to clarify the meaning of hope in palliative nursing, Johnson (2007) identified ten essential attributes of hope:

   (i)   positive expectation—establishing a positive
   (ii) personal qualities—an inner strength
   (iii) spirituality—connections to a higher being

   (iv)   goals—the setting and attainment of short-term goals
   (v)   comfort—being pain free and comfortable
   (vi)   help/caring—behaviors of others such as touch, listening
   (vii) interpersonal relationships—loving relationships with friends and
          family; one's relationships with healthcare providers
   (viii) control—some degree of input and choice regarding care decisions
   (ix)   legacy—leaving behind something of value
   (x)   life review—acknowledgements of past achievements

Johnson's 2007 study also determined the antecedents of hope, those feelings that arise following the realization of the tremendous loss when presented by the diagnosis of the illness: complaints of being physically unwell; possessing some degree of pain and discomfort; given a medical diagnosis of a terminal illness with an uncertain, grave prognosis; faced with depressing facts; described feeling shocked and angry due to the raw fear of death; being in a state of crisis because of the fear of death; feelings of despair, isolation, and abandonment that led to feelings of devaluation of personhood; feeling totally out of control; facing numerous losses and difficult decisions (Johnson, 2007, p. 456). However, the consequences of hope assisted patients to face constructively an uncertain future; to adapt, face mortality, accept their situation. Hope contributed the ability to look beyond pain and to endure and cope with suffering; hope gave patients psychological and physical energy to achieve goals, set priorities, reestablish their faith and spirituality, and to find a desire to keep living; provision of hope facilitated the transcendence of new awareness, enrichment, and a renewed zest for life, enabling patients to appreciate good times and discover reasons for living (Johnson, 2007, pp. 456–7).

   In the context of terminal illness, the concept of hope must be understood differently. In cancer care, especially, the concept of hope is often thought of as the hope of a cure. However, in patients diagnosed with advanced cancer, a cure is not possible, "prolonged survival is doubtful and life may seem anything but hopeful" (McClement & Chochinov, 2008, p. 1169). At the end of life, when science can do no more, the focus of hope changes to one of being, in relationship to loved ones or community. Redefined in this way, hope is borne out in a search for meaning, which appropriately plays out within hospice as opposed to within hospital (Hawthorne & Yurkovich, 2004; Little & Sayers, 2004). Hope plays an important part in a cancer patient's psychosocial and existential well-being, rendering those patients with an enhanced sense of psychospiritual well-being better able to cope with the experience of end-of-life concerns (McClement & Chochinov, 2008). Hope is also viewed as an underlying concept in both dignity and stress and coping in terminally ill patients that enhances their quality of life (Alidina & Tettero, 2010). Conversely, those patients who feel that hope is gone may experience a profound spiritual or existential crisis that can increase the distress and suffering on their physical difficulties.

In face of a diagnosis of life-limiting advanced cancer, patients move through a trajectory of transitions as the illness progresses from one state to another (Clayton et al., 2005). Patients must cope with transitions as the illness progresses and so may pass through a spectrum of hopes: hope for a miracle cure or spontaneous disease remission; hope of living longer than expected; hope in the person's worth as a person and finding meaning in his or her life; hope in the healing of relationships and special times with family/friends; hope in finding spiritual meaning; and hope of a peaceful death (Clayton et al., 2005, pp. 1971–2).

During this time, the physician is charged with the responsibility of communicating critical information and for helping patients to reframe hope (Kiely et al., 2010). Patients want their physicians sensitively to communicate biomedical information; to show care and understanding for their patients as individuals; and to honestly balance realism with hope. Physicians are trained to accomplish this with the "Ask-Tell-Ask" and "Hope for the Best, Prepare for the Worst" techniques, to elicit information about patients' hopes and fears. In the "Ask-Tell-Ask" technique, "the oncologist telling the patient information is bracketed by his asking questions to check that he or she will give the information that is most helpful to the patient" (Evans et al., 2006, p. 421). The approach called "Hope for the Best, Prepare for the Worst" is employed as a way of discussing the possibility of less desirable outcomes with patients, a method that is useful in two ways: "(1) it allows for practical planning while not seeming to take away hopes for a good outcome, and (2) it allows patients to face scary outcomes, which can be the first step toward finding new hopes" (p. 422). The "Hope for the Best, Prepare for the Worst" approach affords multiple possibilities for hopes to be held at the same time, thus facilitating discussions of difficult possibilities that otherwise could not be considered. This represents a step forward for psychosocial progress in patient–clinician communication.

Duggleby et al. conducted a series of studies on hope theory in which elderly terminally ill patients described their worst pain as psychosocial and claimed that they dealt with this pain by maintaining hope. They defined hope as an inner resource that helped them to cope and enhance their quality of life (Duggleby et al., 2007). A grounded hope theory called Transforming Hope emerged in which older palliative patients described hope as "an interrelated, dynamic process of hope, which included acknowledging the reality of their circumstances, searching for meaning, and positive reappraisal" (p. 248). The Transforming Hope theory was used as a basis for a pilot test program of an intervention called the Living with Hope Program (LWHP), which consisted of viewing a research-based film on hope and then, over the course of a week, completing a hope-based activity. The findings suggested that the LWHP group, as opposed to the control group, was effective in raising hope and the quality of life of the elderly terminally ill patients (p. 254).

Related to spirituality is the power of hope and of positive thinking that has shown up in clinical trials as the "placebo effect": that our beliefs are powerful and can positively affect our health outcomes. This led Dr. Herbert Benson to rename the placebo effect as "remembered wellness", which he and Puchalski also noted in the physician–patient relationship as a part of the therapeutic process: positive beliefs about expectations on the part of the patients and on the part of the healthcare professional, and a good relationship between the two parties (Puchalski, 2001, p. 354). Further, Dr. Benson studied the effect of stress on health and implemented the practice of transcendental meditation, which he called the "relaxation response", that proved to be effective therapy for many types of chronic pain.

Living with hope in the presence of a terminal illness entails living in the present, spending quality time with significant others, aiming towards comfort, peace, legacy, and spiritual dimensions. Hope may be characterized as being about "valuing the gift of each day with the positive expectation of a few more good days to follow. Patients review the life they have led and attach meaning to their past achievements, which equates to hope and maximises quality of life" (Johnson, 2007, p. 458). Hope, while subjective, may live in the future: hope for a cure, hope for life over death, or hope for a good death. Hope might be characterized as either part of spirituality or engendering spirituality and meaning. Nevertheless, hope may be seen as a powerful psychosocial coping mechanism that is important to end-of-life care to promote a good death (Benzein et al., 2001), one that "confirms meaning in the dwindling life, with symptoms controlled, dignity preserved, worth recognised and important relationships confirmed" (Little & Sayers, 2004, p. 1336).

6.6 SPIRITUAL COPING AND LIFE REVIEW

> Beyond the inevitable problems of terminal illness, this waning phase of life also encompasses opportunities for life review, life completion and meaningful closure that can profoundly enrich the quality of the person's remaining days—and affect the lives of family members for many years to come.
>
> (Byock, 2000, p. 127)

In contrast to an anticipated death, Byock observed that death by a progressive illness allows time to get one's affairs in order, be they financial or familial. Goodbyes may be said, forgiveness asked for and received, in order to seek and find spiritual strength.

In 1963, Dr. Robert Butler proposed the concept of life review, the use of reminiscence of past experiences, events, and unresolved conflicts structured around certain life. He developed life review as a counseling technique, using it as a means of conflict resolution to help elderly terminal patients prepare for death (Pickrel, 2007). Butler maintained that the processing of past nostalgias or events resulted in self-discovery. Even today, life review is a technique used in group and individual psychotherapy and has been found to be associated with increased life-satisfaction and ego-integrity themes (Holland et al., 2009).

Life review, also termed "reminiscence" or "story-telling", can be a valuable intervention for use with terminal patients. The process of life review provides a means of evaluating and examining where one is and where one may go, in terms of setting goals and resolving conflicts. The life-review process informs the patients' loved ones and caregivers of the scope of past, present, and future concerns of the terminal individual, thereby enabling them to be more understanding and supportive (Pickrel, 2007). The process of life review provides a solution to the potential problem of loss of autonomy encountered by patients at the end of life by conferring some sense of control over life. When a patient's care shifts from cure to comfort, life review can be employed as a valuable intervention in end-of-life care for both patients and caregivers (Jenko et al., 2010).

Randomized controlled trials of a novel psychotherapy, "Short-Term Life Review", by Ando et al. (2010), showed that terminally ill cancer patients who practiced life review therapy improved in both depression and self-esteem scales. The trial of the "Short Term Life Review" intervention confirmed its efficacy to enhance the sense of meaning in terminally ill cancer patients and of its secondary aim to improve its effects on anxiety, depression, and on the elements of a good death (Hope, Burden, Life Completion, and Preparation) (Ando et al., 2010, p. 994). The intervention proved to increase the spiritual well-being of terminally ill cancer patients in facilitating a sense of meaning, alleviating anxiety and depression, and promoting a good death. A major existential concern of cancer patients is the struggle to maintain self-identity, to resist the feeling that the sufferer has become their illness. The implementation of the "Short Term Life Review" protocol allows the building of life stories that incorporate past events into an organized sequence of personal meaning that confirms self-identity and contributes to a feeling of life completion.

Steinhauser et al. (2008, 2009) piloted a study of a version of a life review intervention, called Outlook, to elicit expression of end of life preparation and completion. In the two 2000 research papers published by Steinhauser et al. that defined what constitutes quality at the end of life, patient emotional and spiritual well-being were identified as part of two larger domains, end-of-life preparation and completion (Steinhauser, Christakis et al., 2000; Steinhauser, Clipp et al., 2000). These two areas incorporate both the need for looking back to assess the life lived as well as looking forward to prepare patients and their families for the remaining weeks or months of life. For some terminally ill people, such an evaluation occurs within a traditional religious context; for others it manifests as part of a larger process of meaning making. Nevertheless, the appraisal is facilitated by locating the illness experience in the context of the values and preferences of a whole life. Completion and end-of-life preparation included issues of reviewing life, resolving conflicts, achieving forgiveness, spending time with family and friends, contributing to others, and saying goodbye (Steinhauser et al., 2008, p. 1234).

The Outlook intervention was designed to acknowledge the terminal individual's interruptions of roles, hopes, and plans that the confining gaze of illness can impose and to reacquaint each participant with the entirety of his or her unique life's narrative. The Outlook intervention found that after three weekly interventions of life completion discussions, the terminally ill participants' scores showed a statistically significant decrease of their symptoms of depression in the final months of life.

The Outlook life review intervention is similar in concept to Frankl's logotherapy and shares goals of Chochinov's Dignity Therapy. The intervention is an effort to provide a reproducible and broadly applicable, proactive approach to alleviating emotional, social, and spiritual suffering and to enhancing the quality of life among people approaching the end of life. Outlook introduces the patient to a pattern of "looking back and then orienting forward [that] emphasized that the life trajectory may have been altered but continues" (Steinhauser et al., 2009, p. 402). In line with Dignity Therapy, Outlook appraises the preparation and life completion factors using targeted question during each of three sessions: life story; forgiveness; heritage and legacy (Keall et al., 2011).

The Outlook intervention was also tested in an Australian palliative care setting (Keall et al., 2011), investigating its use in a different cultural setting and was found to be "feasible and acceptable" (p. 458) in that setting. Certain themes were common to both studies, particularly those of regret and forgiveness; participants maintained that they would not change anything in their lives despite hurts or mistakes, as it was their lives.

6.7 SPIRITUALITY AND EXISTENTIAL COPING: THE IMPACT OF THE DIAGNOSIS

> . . . a crack appears in our carefully crafted concept of reality. These existential moments wrench us into a new way of perceiving. They are not simply moments of despair, anxiety, or joy, for, dramatic as those experiences are, we recognize that they are not reality per se, but our response *to* reality. . . . The existential moment, on the other hand, entails a paradigm shift, a jarring, visceral reframing of reality. The very nature of reality is experienced in a new way. We are sucked into the startling realization that the rules of the game are not what we had imagined.

> (Mount, 2003, p. 94)

Boston et al. (2011) performed an integrated literature review on the topic of existential suffering in the palliative care setting. They found little consensus on defining existentialism and existential suffering or how to assess or manage it, other than to say that it is a form of suffering of the dying, difficult to separate out from spirituality, but often conflated with it: "Existential suffering and deep personal anguish at the end of life are some of the most debilitating conditions that occur in patients who are dying, and yet the way we attend to this suffering in their last days is not well understood" (Boston et al., 2011, p. 615). An extensive discussion of existentialism is beyond the scope of this book; instead, an overview of the major concepts involved in this complex topic as they pertain to end-of-life issues—including those variously termed "existential distress", "existential pain", "death anxiety", "death denial", "spiritual pain", "suffering", "demoralization"—are presented.

Existential concerns, apart from physical pain, have been established as an important part of quality of life at the end of life. Cecily Saunders' work on pain management in patients with advanced cancer revealed that suffering was not the only form of pain afflicting dying patients: the consideration of psychological, spiritual, and social factors each became part of her picture of total pain that required treating the entire person (Saunders & Clark, 1999). Understanding the complex, multi-faceted domain of existential concerns that pervades much of the care of the dying presents an enormous challenge, and is largely beyond the scope of this chapter. However, the words describing diverse existential variables indicate the meaning: diminished quality of life, social isolation, anxiety, suffering, distress (physical and emotional), depression, pain, desire for hastened death, hopelessness, burden to others, loss of dignity, meaning and purpose, despair, angst, demoralization, helplessness, hopelessness (LeMay & Wilson, 2008). Speaking about the results of a 2005 study, Chochinov et al. (2005) posited that "when a broad range of influences are considered concurrently, existential issues emerge most prominently" (p. 10).

Kissane (2000, in Lee et al., 2006, p. 291) defined existential distress as "the state of an individual confronting his or her own mortality that arises from feelings of powerlessness, disappointment, futility, meaninglessness, remorse, death anxiety, and disruption with his or her engagement with and purpose in life" that appears to be a ubiquitous part of the end-stage cancer experience. The term "existential distress" also refers to what has been called death anxiety (Pyszczynski et al., 1999). Existential distress is a construct separate from general anxiety, depression, somatic distress, and global psychological distress (Lichtenthal et al., 2009) and correlates with time since diagnosis and closeness to death (Weisman & Worden, 1976–77; Lichtenthal et al., 2009; Lee, 2008). Death anxiety has been found to interfere with the achievement of a peaceful death (Bolmsjo, 2000; Benito et al., 2013).

Existential concerns may be addressed with mechanisms of meaning-making coping. The existential concept of spirituality entails the need to find satisfactory answers to questions about the meaning of life, illness, and death, although existentialism may or may not involve belief in a higher being or in an organized religion (Breitbart, 2001). Puchalski highlighted the markers of a person experiencing existential suffering: lack of meaning; questioning meaning about one's own existence; concerns about afterlife; questioning the meaning of suffering; and seeking spiritual assistance (Puchalski, 2012, p. iii51).

Miller et al. (2005) designed an intervention that emphasized the psychosocial-spiritual aspects of living and dying and offered strategies for living well despite life-threatening illnesses. The intervention is known as the Supportive-Affective Group Experience for Persons with Life-Threatening Illness (LTI-SAGE). The group process was defined as adult affective education and support, not therapy. The underlying purpose of LTI-SAGE was for each group member to develop a greater sense of hope, courage, and connection. The process relied heavily on discussing experiences, expressing feelings, and sharing support, and included topics of spirituality. The results of this randomized trial indicated qualified support for the efficacy of LTI-SAGE in reducing depression symptoms, increasing spiritual well-being, and reducing death-related feelings of meaninglessness.

Quality of life in the palliative care setting and throughout the disease trajectory in cancer patients is associated with and determined by the existential or spiritual domains (Cohen et al., 1996). Whereas reactions to the diagnosis of cancer range from normative awareness to demoralization, often the diagnosis is automatically considered a death sentence, replete with pain, suffering, and disfigurement. Cancer remains the most feared diagnosis and is not culturally dependent, as evidenced by studies on the "existential plight" from many countries such as Australia, Britain, Japan, Sweden, Norway, and Israel (Lee, 2008, p. 781).

Weisman and Worden's (1976–77) classic study of the "existential plight of cancer", an expression they coined, described the poorly recognized but significant period that starts with the diagnosis and continues through the first one hundred days. This period of two to three months is "not a mere metaphor, but a distinct phase of cancer to which almost all patients are subjected. Quite literally, it is a luckless predicament in which one's very existence seems endangered" (Weisman & Worden, 1976–77, p. 3). With disease progression, vulnerability increases, but at the time of diagnosis, psychosocial distress enabled the investigators to predict within limits which patients would cope effectively and which would fail to do so. Whereas the existential plight is a common phenomenon, variations exist in the levels of distress that are associated with thoughts about one's mortality and purpose in life.

Existential distress in patients at the end of life presents as demoralization, with symptoms of hopelessness and helplessness caused by a lack of meaning and purpose in life and is a common occurrence that Kissane, in 2001, has termed as the "demoralization syndrome" (in Robinson et al., 2015). The demoralization syndrome comprises symptoms of hopelessness and helplessness caused by a loss of purpose and meaning in life that spans a "spectrum of mental states, from a mild loss of confidence—'disheartenment,' to the beginning of losing hope and purpose—'despondency,' to a state in which all hope is lost—'despair,' through to severe demoralization where meaning and purpose are lost" (Robinson et al., 2015, pp. 595–6). Demoralization is a significant mental health concern because it has been associated with a desire for hastened death. Demoralization is a treatable condition that has been differentiated from depression, which is characterized by a loss of anticipatory pleasure, and is seen to potentiate suicidal ideation.

Kissane (2012) embroidered upon Yalom's original concepts of the existential struggle by specifying that the major forms of existential challenge include

> (1) death anxiety, (2) loss and change, (3) freedom which involves choices, responsibility, and guilt, (4) dignity of the self, (5) isolation/fundamental aloneness, representing the gulf between the self and others, (6) altered quality of relationships, (7) lack of meaning which impels individuals to create personal meaning; and (8) mystery.
>
> (Kissane, 2012, p. 1502)

The forms of distress, specifically those of dignity and meaning, have been approached clinically with psychosocial interventions for improving end-of-life care and promoting a good death.

For some patients, salience of mortality, symptom burden, and fear of the future present as death distress, whereas for others, awareness of mortality presents an opportunity for adaptive value that can change one's life priorities. Existential or death awareness presents a paradox that lies in its potential to be both psychologically paralyzing as well as instrumental in mobilizing a tenacious will to live (Lee & Loiselle, 2012). A diagnosis of cancer can trigger existential awareness, the contemplation of mortality, personal identity, autonomy, dignity, life meaning and purpose, and connections with others within the context of life and death (Frankl, 1966; Bolmsjo, 2000). However, existential awareness in those with advanced cancer who have an accurate prognostic awareness does not necessarily suffer existential distress (Blinderman & Cherny, 2005).

Yang et al. (2010) discussed the nature and characteristics of an existential crisis that was demonstrated in a grounded, qualitative study that cited the following elements:

> Acute awareness of one's own finitude; dissolving of the future appears alarming; a loss of meaning causes disruption in the lifeline; experience of fear, anxiety, panic, despair; loneliness caused by the event;

powerlessness in relation to the course of illness and one's ability to deal with one's own intense emotions; identity crisis.

(Yang et al., 2010, pp. 58–9)

A diagnosis of a life-limiting illness is an event that profoundly disturbs a patient's normal functioning. The knowledge of impending death creates an existential crisis wherein life's meaning must be reassessed because the usual objective coping strategies have been rendered void. Subjective meaning must be sought and spirituality struggled with daily, in a new "life-as-it-is" assumption (Yang et al., 2010, p. 57). Those patients who allowed the reality of impending death into their consciousness and lived through the emotions dealt with the existential crisis by giving in to the mourning process. Thereby, they were able to abandon the familiar framework of their old meanings and became able to connect to the present moment (Yang et al., 2010). Thus, clinicians need to understand that when they inform a patient of a terminal diagnosis, they are impacting on that patient's existential domain:

> The fundamental relevance of existential concerns to the patient's experience of illness, the caregiver's important opportunity to lend support and act as a catalyst for coping, and the need to ensure that these issues are addressed must therefore be considered integral components of competent care in oncology.
>
> (Cohen et al., 1996, p. 582)

The success of modern disease management effected a paradoxical potential for existential distress and suffering wherein patients question what their death will be like and when it will occur.

Comprehending the factors that underlie existential concerns at the end of life is the focus of a sizable body of research. Some studies concluded that for patients suffering with a terminal illness, existential concerns can increase their risk for suicidal ideation and desire for hastened death that are then seen as a good death. Other studies have established existential concerns as an important dimension of quality of life at the end of life, easing a path to a good death. Mount et al. (2007) explained the quality of life continuum as a dialectic that extends from suffering and anguish at one extreme, representing wounding, to an experience of integrity and wholeness at the other, representing healing. This 2007 study discusses the "healing connection" that places the individual within a larger context that in turn supports meaning, self-esteem, and quality of life. Mount posited an influence of the teachings of wisdom traditions regarding the importance to healing of: acceptance of self and one's present reality; identifying, and opting for, what is still possible within the constraints of present circumstances; coming into the present moment; and letting go of the need for control and ruminations about past and future; and that "acceptance of this nature is the transcendent alternative to denial" (p. 385).

Existentialist thinkers, such as Frankl, view suffering as a potential spring-board, both for having a need for meaning and for finding it (Greenstein & Breitbart, 2000, p. 487). When the inevitability of one's own death is made clear with receipt of a cancer diagnosis, existential awareness is triggered by thoughts of life and death, life's meaning and purpose, and connections with loved ones (Frankl, 1966; Bolmsjo, 2000). Diagnosed patients often manifest denial as a common defense mechanism in the emotional adjustment to cancer. Prognostic denial can help protect the terminally ill from feelings of death anxiety, allowing them to "titrate reality at a pace they feel tolerable" (Chochinov et al., 2000, p. 502). Feelings of distress can be alleviated by an increase in meaning and sense of purpose, despite traumatic causes or because of them, and may increase the quality of life of terminal patients (Greenstein & Breitbart, 2000). Patients who found a greater sense of meaning in life experienced more enjoyment in life, even in the case of severe pain (Brady et al., 1999).

Supportive psycho-existential interventions have been developed to alleviate despair in patients and families that include components that directly address these needs. One intervention (Cole & Pargament, 1999) explored existential concerns within the participants' spiritual frameworks, enhanced spiritual coping and resolved spiritual struggle and strain, and appeared to offer benefits in terms of preventing problems with pain and depression. The study by Morita et al. (2004) categorized the existential concerns of Japanese terminally ill cancer patients as "relationship-related concerns, loss of control, burden on others, loss of continuity, uncompleted life task, hope/hopelessness, and acceptance/preparation" (p. 137). A study involving a brief existential intervention, the Life Tape Project (LTP), was created to harness and bolster family support and understanding (Rosenbaum et al., 2006; Garlan et al., 2010). LTP yielded broad, positive psychosocial changes for participants, providing intervention-specific benefits, especially in the areas of symbolic immortality (passing on personal values and philosophy), self-reflection and growth, and improved family cohesion and communication. Participants, especially those who had perceived their cancer as a "threat of death, and responded with intense fear or helplessness, also reported more general reductions in mood disturbance, improvements in aspects of well-being (including overall quality of life), satisfaction with the understanding they received, and enhanced cancer related posttraumatic growth" (Garlan et al., 2010, p. 244). Not only reporting significant improvement in physical well-being, the aspect of social support—feeling seen and heard—proved valuable in combating existential isolation, a factor proven by a number of other studies investigating factors associated with interviewing patients in various stages of terminality (Emanuel et al., 2004). Feeling seen and heard is a major component in cited aspects of good dying, such as personhood, dignity, spirituality, life review, legacy, and hope.

6.8 SPIRITUALITY AND MEANING-MAKING COPING: FROM DIAGNOSIS TO DEATH

> Patients facing a serious illness or the end of life may experience numerous spiritual concerns. Some of the most common include an inability to find meaning and purpose, hopelessness, anger at God, asking Why? and struggling with a will to live.
>
> (Borneman et al., 2010)

Clinical research has provided support for adopting the biopsychosocial-spiritual model of quality of life assessment in clinical practice, largely in oncology but also in other areas such as Chronic Kidney Disease (Davison & Jhangri, 2013). Mounting evidence suggests that spiritual well-being is in fact a crucial, unique, core domain to be considered when attempting to determine a patient's actual QOL following diagnosis of a life-threatening illness (Breitbart et al., 2004; Walter, 1997; Whitford & Olver, 2012). Likewise, the importance of meaning and peace at times of stress, such as a dire diagnosis, are factors associated with coping styles that may go on to impact patients' survival times and other domains of QOL such as physical and functional well-being. The literature reflects substantial qualitative and empirical evidence to suggest that the ability to reconstruct a sense of meaning following a diagnosis of cancer is related to important psychosocial outcomes such as improved self-esteem, greater optimism, and less psychological distress (Lee & Cohen, 2004).

The Foundations of Spirituality and Meaning at the End of Life

> In the nexus between cognitive reasoning and personal feeling lies the realm of meaning.
>
> (Breitbart et al., 2004, p. 367)

Prior to a diagnosis of cancer—or to the occurrence/onset of a life-limiting illness—one's belief system provided some type of stability and security; however, such a diagnosis or event often launches a search for meaning, motivated by the existential plight, during which most patients seek to appraise the impact of cancer (Lee, 2008). The "existential plight of cancer" refers to the search for meaning following a cancer experience, in which a key determinant of overall quality of life is global meaning, defined as the general sense that one's life has order and purpose (Lee, 2008). Individuals with diagnoses of life-limiting illnesses benefit from a new integration of the meaning of the illness into their lives, with efforts to facilitate an exploration of meaning making (Lee & Loiselle, 2012). Depending upon one's life schema or personal motivation being more allied to spirituality or to religion, individual variations and degrees of the process of the search to make meaning commences.

Viktor Frankl saw meaning as a fundamental drive in human psychology; the need to find a sense of meaning, purpose, and value in life forms a spiritual component of the human experience (Breitbart & Heller, 2003). Meaning may be defined in terms of one's relatedness to or perceptions of significant aspects of one's life and experience, of one's self, both bodily and psychically (Chochinov, 2003). Meaning can be gained despite the diagnosis of a life-limiting disease, but it may also be lessened or lost, depending on how one views the world. Meaning-making coping is characterized by a necessary but distressing confrontation with loss that, if followed by a plan to fulfill a purpose and order in life, can lead to improved psychological well-being and lessening of psychological distress (Lee et al., 2006).

Meaning is a multidimensional existential construct operationally defined as comprising different levels: *global* meaning, encompassing an individual's enduring beliefs and valued goals such as those one bears prior to a cancer diagnosis (That which in my life has meaning and purpose); *situational* meaning, or meaning that is formed in the interaction between global meaning and the circumstances of a particular person–environment transaction (Park & Folkman, 1997, p. 116) such as that associated with a cancer diagnosis (Why me?); and *existential* meaning, or the meaning of life in general (What is the meaning of life and death?). Conversely, an absence of meaning, or the presence of a pessimistic outlook, could lead to despair or to demoralization (Park & Folkman, 1997; Lee & Cohen, 2004; Henry et al., 2010). The distinction between global meaning and situational meaning allows distinguishing among different types of situational meaning, including appraised meaning, the search for meaning (meaning-making coping), and meaning as outcome (changes in global meaning) (Park & Folkman, 1997, p. 132). Park and Folkman (1997) defined meaning making as the "eventual integration of situational meaning with global meaning through cognitive reappraisals of both the appraised meaning of the situation and global beliefs and goals" (p. 132).

The emergence of palliative care and its emphasis on pain management in end-of-life care allowed inclusion of person-centered goals of care. Spiritual well-being and the search for meaning became important resources for coping with emotional and existential concerns as patients neared death. Spiritual well-being and a sense of meaning have been shown to have beneficial effects on terminally ill individuals (Brady et al., 1999) and to bear a strong negative effect on hopelessness, depression, despair, suicidal ideation, and desire for hastened death. Thus, the development of psychosocial interventions that support a focus on increasing and/or maintaining a sense of meaning and purpose became an important priority in palliative end-of-life care (Breitbart, 2001; Breitbart & Heller, 2003; Breitbart et al., 2004).

Novel Modalities Integrating Meaning and Spirituality into End-of-Life Care

A qualitative study of a meaning-based coping approach by Lethborg et al. (2008) explored how patients facing a life-limiting illness or impending death from cancer experienced meaning and how they applied meaning to cope with the diagnosis. Meaning may be gained or lost in such situations, depending upon how an individual behaves according to a basic system of beliefs or concepts that have developed over time. These notions facilitate the ways in which we function effectively by providing expectations about ourselves and the world. This conceptual system is represented by a set of assumptions that have proven, over time, to be personally practicable as we deal with the world. In face of negative life events, such as a diagnosis of life-threatening illness or of impending death, we feel vulnerable and disbe-lieving that such an event could occur in our world: the assumptions sup-porting this sense of invulnerability would be among the most fundamental postulates in our assumptive world (Janoff-Bulman, 1989, p. 117). One's world, as it has been heretofore known, is apt no longer to feel safe. Also, the way in which the patient then appraises the situation presented by the diagnosis influences the experience. A balance prevails if one is able to main-tain psychological stability in the face of stressful events by processing the situation to gain a sense of coherence, a concept attributed to Antonovsky (1987, in Lethborg et al., 2008, p. 29). Meaning-based coping describes the role of meaning individuals use to reappraise their situation and to realize a better resolution with their world view. The information produced by the study participants revealed three interrelated domains: the first domain was associated with the concept of assumptive world and involves experience living with advanced cancer with its attendant isolation and fear of death; the sense of loss of people and life goals; and fear of a foreshortened life. The second domain, associated with sense of coherence, was marked by an attempt to live without entirely focusing on having cancer. The third domain was involved with meaning-based coping wherein patients committed to making the most of the time left to them. The interrelationship of the three domains presents an integrated model reflective of the lived experiences of patients coping with advanced cancer with meaning-based coping.

Lee et al. (2006) developed and piloted the Meaning Making intervention (MMi), a novel approach to exploring existential issues in an ambulatory care setting based on the insights of the participants with cancer undergoing treatment. The findings suggested that a greater sense of security to cope with an uncertain future emerged and levels of self-esteem and self-efficacy improved. The MMi was tested by Lee in 2008, using an exercise, Life-line, based on three tasks to be completed by the patient and clinician. The first task is to acknowledge the present, in which the patient is encouraged to tell their story; the second task encourages acknowledging the past, in which patients are encouraged to talk about pivotal life events that occurred prior to their diagnosis of cancer; the third task is to live in the present for the future, in which patients are encouraged to talk about how to live life as fully as possible in the context of cancer. Such creative, evidence-based approaches like the MMi are necessary to facilitate a dialog with patients so that quality of life, not always the treatment and management of the illness, becomes one of the guiding forces in their search for meaning following cancer (Lee, 2008, p. 784).

6.9 PSYCHOLOGICAL UNDERPINNINGS OF SPIRITUALITY

> Patients frequently convey various concerns about death and the manner in which they will die. They often imagine that their suffering will be overwhelming and that in the face of such suffering, their health care team will be rendered helpless. Exploring the specifics of these concerns and providing explicit information about symptom management can provide patients with tremendous comfort and relief. . . . Psychiatrists can play a role in facilitating the appropriate grief work and can often assist patients who search for a continued sense of purpose and meaning in the face of imminent death.
>
> (Chochinov, 2000, p. 144.)

As the needs of terminally ill patients became better understood, end-of-life measures were refocused and expanded beyond symptom control to include psychiatric, existential, and spiritual domains of psychosocial care (Breitbart et al., 2004). The "psych" part of the biopsychosocial-spiritual model of end-of-life spiritual care in palliative medicine began to attract the focus of mental health researchers. Dying patients experience various symptoms as death draws near and the distinction between somatic distress and psychological or spiritual disquietude becomes less clear. Patients nearing death face enormous psychological challenges and the psychiatrist working in this setting must be sensitive to these issues and prepared to explore them in depth. Psychiatrists are in a particularly advantageous position to assist dying patients, their families, and care providers in navigating this challenging terrain: their knowledge of physical medicine in combination with a broad range of psychiatric expertise creates a rich set of skills and informs the understanding of palliative medicine and the multiple facets of caring for the dying (Chochinov, 2000, p. 143).

Working with terminal cancer patients during the decade of physician-assisted suicide, euthanasia, and suicidal ideation, as well as with HIV/AIDS patients, psychiatric oncologists grasped the need, not merely for relief of suffering of physical pain, but also for the relief of psychological symptoms and of existential distress (Chochinov, 2000; Greenstein & Breitbart, 2000; Breitbart, 2001). The most common sources of psychological and psychiatric suffering for patients are anxiety and depressive and cognitive disorders (Jacobsen & Breitbart, 1996). Thus, psychiatric morbidity at the end of life can be significant and cause severe, but potentially remediable, pain and suffering to terminally ill patients and their families.

Quality care for the psychiatric complications of terminal illness should be an integral component of excellent, comprehensive end-of-life care, in order to promote a good death. The preeminent task of dying for patients and families at the end of life is that of loss: loss of self-esteem due to the disabilities of the illness and loss of the patient that shatters the relationship between the patient and the family. Grief is the painful, normative response to loss, so that the physician must differentiate between a normal coping response and pathologic responses. Psychiatric morbidity in this setting is very high, partly because psychiatric symptoms at the end of life are viewed as normal parts of the dying process. However, such symptoms respond to treatment (Shuster et al., 1999, p. 1; Block, 2001, p. 2898). Good psychiatric end-of-life care requires psychological and spiritual assessment of patients with life-limiting illnesses. Only when the physician has evaluated physical discomfort and possible dysfunctional responses to the patient's imminent death, can that patient be assisted toward having a good death. The normative psychiatric desires of patients seeking a good death are:

1. Patients facing death are concerned with optimizing physical comfort.
2. A terminal patient's ability to feel like him/herself, despite the illness, enables and reflects good coping.
3. Relationships are changed by terminal illness: to connect more deeply often wars with the physical dependency that fosters fear of being a burden or of being abandoned.
4. The desire for making meaning of one's life involves legacy and leave-taking.
5. Patients often seek a sense of control over how they die.
6. Preparing for death may entail financial details, planning the funeral, and what to expect of the process of dying (adapted from Block, 2001, pp. 2900–3).

CITATIONS: CHAPTER 6

Alidina, K., & Tettero, I. (2010). Exploring the therapeutic value of hope in palliative nursing. *Palliative & Supportive Care, 8*(3), 353–358. http://doi.org/10.1017/S1478951510000155.

Ando, M., Morita, T., Akechi, T., & Okamoto, T. (2010). Efficacy of short-term life-review interviews on the spiritual well-being of terminally ill cancer patients. *Journal of Pain and Symptom Management, 39*(6), 993–1002. http://doi.org/10.1016/j.jpainsymman.2009.11.320.

Ando, M., Morita, T., Lee, V., & Okamoto, T. (2008). A pilot study of transformation, attributed meanings to the illness, and spiritual well-being for terminally ill cancer patients. *Palliative & Supportive Care, 6*(4), 335–340. http://doi.org/10.1017/S1478951508000539.

Ardelt, M., Landes, S.D., Gerlach, K.R., & Fox, L.P. (2013). Rediscovering internal strengths of the aged: The beneficial impact of wisdom, mastery, purpose in life, and spirituality on aging well. In J.D. Sinnott (Ed.), *Positive Psychology* (pp. 97–119). New York: Springer. http://doi.org/10.1007/978-1-4614-7282-7.

Astrow, A.B., Wexler, A., Texeira, K., He, M.K., & Sulmasy, D.P. (2007). Is failure to meet spiritual needs associated with cancer patients' perceptions of quality of care and their satisfaction with care? *Journal of Clinical Oncology: Official Journal of the American Society of Clinical Oncology, 25*(36), 5753–5757. http://doi.org/10.1200/JCO.2007.12.4362.

Balboni, M. J., Sullivan, A., Amobi, A., Phelps, A. C., Gorman, D. P., Zollfrank, A., . . . Balboni, T. A. (2013). Why is spiritual care infrequent at the end of life? Spiritual care perceptions among patients, nurses, and physicians and the role of training. *Journal of Clinical Oncology: Official Journal of the American Society of Clinical Oncology, 31*(4), 461–467. http://doi.org/10.1200/JCO.2012.44.6443.

Balboni, T. A., Balboni, M., Enzinger, A. C., Gallivan, K., Paulk, M. E., Wright, A. A., . . . Prigerson, H. G. (2013). Provision of spiritual support to patients with advanced cancer by religious communities and associations with medical care at the end of life. *JAMA Internal Medicine, 173*(12), 1109–1117. http://doi.org/10.1001/jamainternmed.2013.903.

Balboni, T. A., Balboni, M. J., Paulk, M. E., Phelps, A. C., Wright, A. A., Peteet, J., . . . Prigerson, H. (2011). Support of cancer patients' spiritual needs and associations with medical care costs at the end of life. *Cancer, 117*(23), 5383–5391. http://doi.org/10.1002/cncr.26221.

Balboni, T. A., Paulk, M. E., Balboni, M. J., Phelps, A. C., Loggers, E. T., Wright, A. A., . . . Prigerson, H. G. (2010). Provision of spiritual care to patients with advanced cancer: Associations with medical care and quality of life near death. *Journal of Clinical Oncology, 28*(3). http://doi.org/10.1200/JCO.2009.24.8005.

Balboni, T. A., Vanderwerker, L. C., Block, S. D., Paulk, M. E., Lathan, C. S., Peteet, J. R., & Prigerson, H. G. (2007). Religiousness and spiritual support among advanced cancer patients and associations with end-of-life treatment preferences and quality of life. *Journal of Clinical Oncology: Official Journal of the American Society of Clinical Oncology, 25*(5), 555–560. http://doi.org/10.1200/JCO.2006.07.9046.

Benito, E., Oliver, A., Galiana, L., Barreto, P., Pascual, A., Gomis, C., & Barbero, J. (2013). Development and validation of a new tool for the assessment and spiritual care of palliative care patients. *Journal of Pain and Symptom Management.* 47(6): 1008–1018. http://doi.org/10.1016/j.jpainsymman.2013.06.018.

Benzein, E., Norberg, A., & Saveman, B. I. (2001). The meaning of the lived experience of hope in patients with cancer in palliative home care. *Palliative Medicine, 15*(2), 117–126. http://doi.org/10.1191/026921601675617254.

Best, M., Butow, P., & Olver, I. (2014). Spiritual support of cancer patients and the role of the doctor. *Supportive Care in Cancer: Official Journal of the Multinational Association of Supportive Care in Cancer, 22*(5), 1333–1339. http://doi.org/10.1007/s00520-013-2091-1.

Blinderman, C. D., & Cherny, N. I. (2005). Existential issues do not necessarily result in existential suffering: Lessons from cancer patients in Israel. *Palliative Medicine, 19*(5), 371–380. Retrieved from www.ncbi.nlm.nih.gov/pubmed/16111060.

Block, S. (2001). Psychological considerations, growth, and transcendence at the end of life: The art of the possible. *JAMA: The Journal of the American Medical Association, 285*(22), 2898–2906. Retrieved from www.ncbi.nlm.nih.gov/pubmed/11743842.

Bolmsjo, I. (2000). Existential issues in palliative care—Interviews with cancer patients. *Journal of Palliative Care, 16*(2), 20–24.

Borneman, T., Ferrell, B., & Puchalski, C. M. (2010). Evaluation of the FICA Tool for spiritual assessment. *Journal of Pain and Symptom Management, 40*(2), 163–173. http://doi.org/10.1016/j.jpainsymman.2009.12.019.

Boston, P., Bruce, A., & Schreiber, R. (2011). Existential suffering in the palliative care setting: An integrated literature review. *Journal of Pain and Symptom Management, 41*(3), 604–618. http://doi.org/10.1016/j.jpainsymman.2010.05.010.

Brady, M. J., Peterman, A. H., Fitchett, G., Mo, M., & Cella, D. (1999). A case for including spirituality in quality of life measurement in oncology. *Psycho-Oncology, 8*(5), 417–428. Retrieved from www.ncbi.nlm.nih.gov/pubmed/10559801.

Breitbart, W. (1999). Physician-assisted suicide: The influence of psychosocial issues. In E. Chochinov, M. Harvey, & W. Breitbart (Eds.), *Handbook of psychiatry in palliative medicine* (pp. 357–373). Cary, NC: Oxford University Press.

Breitbart, W. (2001). Spirituality and meaning in supportive care: Spirituality- and meaning-centered group psychotherapy interventions in advanced cancer. *Supportive Care in Cancer: Official Journal of the Multinational Association of Supportive Care in Cancer, 10*(4), 272–280, published online. http://doi.org/10.1007/s005200100289.

Breitbart, W., Gibson, C., Poppito, S. R. (2004). Psychotherapeutic interventions at the end of life: A focus on meaning and spirituality. *Canadian Journal of Psychiatry, 49*(6), 366–73.

Breitbart, W., & Heller, K. S. (2003). Reframing hope: Meaning-centered care for patients near the end of life. *Journal of Palliative Medicine, 6*(6), 979–988.

Breitbart, W., & Rosenfeld, B. D. (1999). Physician-assisted suicide: The influence of psychosocial issues. *Cancer Control, 6*(2), 146–161.

Breitbart, W., Rosenfeld, B., Pessin, H., Applebaum, A., Kulikowski, J., & Lichtenthal, W. G. (2015). Meaning-centered group psychotherapy: An effective intervention for improving psychological well-being in patients with advanced cancer. *Journal of Clinical Oncology: Official Journal of the American Society of Clinical Oncology, 33*(7), 749–754. http://doi.org/10.1200/JCO.2014.57.2198.

Byock, I. (1996). The nature of suffering and the nature of opportunity at the end of life. *Clinics in Geriatric Medicine, 12*(2), 237–252.

Byock, I. (2000). Completing the continuum of cancer care: Integrating life-prolongation and palliation. *CA: A Cancer Journal for Clinicians, 50*(2), 123–132. Retrieved from www.ncbi.nlm.nih.gov/pubmed/10870488.

Chibnall, J. T., Videen, S. D., Duckro, P. N., & Miller, D. K. (2002). Psychosocial-spiritual correlates of death distress in patients with life-threatening medical conditions. *Palliative Medicine, 16*(4), 331–338. http://doi.org/10.1191/0269216302pm544oa.

Chochinov, H. M. (2000). Psychiatry & terminal illness. *Canadian Journal of Psychiatry, 45*, 143–150.

Chochinov, H. M. (2003). Thinking outside the box: Depression, hope, and meaning at the end of life. *Journal of Palliative Medicine, 6*(6), 973–977.

Chochinov, H. M., & Cann, B. J. (2005). Interventions to enhance the spiritual aspects of dying. *Journal of Palliative Medicine, 8*(Suppl. 1), S103–S115. http://doi.org/10.1089/jpm.2005.8.s-103.

Chochinov, H. M., Hack, T., Hassard, T., Kristjanson, L. J., McClement, S. E., & Harlos, M. (2005). Understanding the will to live in patients nearing death. *Psychosomatics, 46*(1), 7–10. http://doi.org/10.1176/appi.psy.46.1.7.

Chochinov, H. M., Tataryn, D. J., Wilson, K. G., Enns, M., & Lander, S. (2000). Prognostic awareness and the terminally ill. *Psychosomatics, 41*(6), 500–504. http://doi.org/10.1176/appi.psy.41.6.500.

Clayton, J. M., Butow, P. N., Arnold, R. M., & Tattersall, M. H. N. (2005). Fostering coping and nurturing hope when discussing the future with terminally ill cancer patients and their caregivers. *Cancer, 103*(9), 1965–1975. http://doi.org/10.1002/cncr.21011.

Cohen A. B., & Koenig, H. G. (2003). Religiosity and spirituality in the biopsychosocial model of health and ageing. *Ageing International, 28*(3), 215–241.

Cohen, S. R., Boston, P., Mount, B., & Porterfield, P. (2001). Changes in quality of life following admission to palliative care units. *Palliative Medicine, 15*(5), 363–371. http://doi.org/10.1191/026921601680419401.

Cohen, S. R., Mount, B. M., Tomas, J.J.N., & Mount, L. F. (1996). Existential well-being is an important determinant of quality of life. *Cancer, 77*(3), 576–586.

Cole, B., & Pargament, K. (1999). Re-creating your life: A spiritual/psychotherapeutic intervention for people diagnosed with cancer. *Psycho-Oncology*, 8(5), 395–407. Retrieved from www.ncbi.nlm.nih.gov/pubmed/10559799.

Coward, D. D., & Reed, P. (1996). Self-transcendence: A resource for healing at the end of life. *Issues in Mental Health Nursing*, 17, 275–288.

Daaleman, T. P., & VandeCreek, L. (2000). Placing religion and spirituality in end-of-life care. *JAMA: The Journal of the American Medical Association*, 284(19), 2514–2517.

Davison, S., & Jhangri, G. S. (2013). The relationship between spirituality, psychosocial adjustment to illness and health-related quality of life in patients with advanced chronic kidney disease. *Journal of Pain and Symptom Management*, 45(2), 170–178. http://doi.org/10.1016/j.jpainsymman.2012.02.019.

Delgado-Guay, M. O. (2014). Spirituality and religiosity in supportive and palliative care. *Current Opinion in Supportive and Palliative Care*, 8(3), 308–313. http://doi.org/10.1097/SPC.0000000000000079.

Delgado-Guay, M. O., Hui, D., Parsons, H. A., Govan, K., De la Cruz, M., Thorney, S., & Bruera, E. (2011). Spirituality, religiosity, and spiritual pain in advanced cancer patients. *Journal of Pain and Symptom Management*, 41(6), 986–994. http://doi.org/10.1016/j.jpainsymman.2010.09.017.

Duggleby, W. D., Degner, L., Williams, A., Wright, K., Cooper, D., Popkin, D., & Holtslander, L. (2007). Living with hope: Initial evaluation of a psychosocial hope intervention for older palliative home care patients. *Journal of Pain and Symptom Management*, 33(3), 247–257. http://doi.org/10.1016/j.jpainsymman.2006.09.013.

Duggleby, W. D., Ghosh, S., Cooper, D., & Dwernychuk, L. (2013). Hope in newly diagnosed cancer patients. *Journal of Pain and Symptom Management*, 46(5), 661–670. http://doi.org/10.1016/j.jpainsymman.2012.12.004.

Efficace, F., & Marrone, R. (2002). Spiritual issues and quality of life assessment in cancer care. *Death Studies*, 26(9), 743–756. http://doi.org/10.1080/07481180290106526.

Eliott, J. A., & Olver, I. N. (2009). Hope, life, and death: A qualitative analysis of dying cancer patients' talk about hope. *Death Studies*, 33(7), 609–638. http://doi.org/10.1080/07481180903011982.

Emanuel, E. J., Fairclough, D. L., Wolfe, P., & Emanuel, L. (2004). Talking with terminally ill patients and their caregivers about death, dying, and bereavement. *Archives of Internal Medicine*, 164(18), 1999–2004. Retrieved from http://archinte.jamanetwork.com/pdfaccess.ashx?ResourceID=1299857&PDFSource=13.

Epstein-Peterson, Z. D., Sullivan, A. J., Enzinger, A. C., Trevino, K. M., Zollfrank, A. A., Balboni, M. J., . . . Balboni, T. A. (2014). Examining forms of spiritual care provided in the advanced cancer setting. *The American Journal of Hospice & Palliative Care*, e-pub ahead, 1–8. http://doi.org/10.1177/1049909114540318.

Evans, W. G., Tulsky, J. A., Back, A. L., & Arnold, R. M. (2006). Communication at times of transitions: How to help patients cope with loss and re-define hope. *Cancer Journal (Sudbury, Mass.)*, 12(5), 417–424. Retrieved from www.ncbi.nlm.nih.gov/pubmed/17034677.

Frankl, V. E. (1966). Self-transcendence as a human phenomenon. *Journal of Humanistic Psychology*, 6, 97–106.

Frankl, V. E. (1984). *Man's search for meaning* (third edition). New York: Pocket Books.

Garlan, R. W., Butler, L. D., Rosenbaum, E., Siegel, A., & Spiegel, D. (2010). Perceived benefits and psychosocial outcomes of a brief existential family intervention for cancer patients/survivors. *OMEGA—Journal of Death and Dying*, 62(3), 243–268. http://doi.org/10.2190/OM.62.3.c.

Gonzalez, P., Castañeda, S. F., Dale, J., Medeiros, E. A., Buelna, C., Nuñez, A., . . . Talavera, G. A. (2014). Spiritual well-being and depressive symptoms among cancer survivors. *Supportive Care in Cancer: Official Journal of the Multinational Association of Supportive Care in Cancer, 22*(9), 2393–2400. http://doi.org/10.1007/s00520-014-2207-2.

Greenstein, M., & Breitbart, W. (2000). Cancer and the experience of meaning: A group psychotherapy program for people with cancer. *American Journal of Psychotherapy, 54*, 486–500.

Hawthorne, D. L., & Yurkovich, N. J. (2004). Hope at the end of life: Making a case for hospice. *Palliative & Supportive Care, 2*(4), 415–7. Retrieved from www.ncbi.nlm.nih.gov/pubmed/16594405.

Henry, M., Cohen, S. R., Lee, V., Sauthier, P., Provencher, D., Drouin, P., . . . Mayo, N. (2010). The Meaning-Making intervention (MMi) appears to increase meaning in life in advanced ovarian cancer: A randomized controlled pilot study. *Psycho-Oncology, 19*(12), 1340–1347. http://doi.org/10.1002/pon.1764.

Holland, J., Poppito, S., Nelson, C., Weiss, T., Greenstein, M., Martin, A., . . . Roth, A. (2009). Reappraisal in the eighth life cycle stage: A theoretical psychoeducational intervention in elderly patients with cancer. *Palliative & Supportive Care, 7*(3), 271–279. http://doi.org/10.1017/S1478951509990198.

Jacobsen, P. B., & Breitbart, W. (1996). Psychosocial aspects of palliative care. *Cancer Control, 3*, 214–222.

Janoff-Bulman, R. (1989). Assumptive worlds and the stress of traumatic events: Applications of the schema construct. *Social Cognition, 7*(2), 113–136.

Jenko, M., Gonzalez, L., & Alley, P. (2010). Life review in critical care: Possibilities at the end of life. *Critical Care Nurse, 30*(1), 17–27; quiz 28. http://doi.org/10.4037/ccn2010122.

Johnson, S. (2007). Hope in terminal illness: An evolutionary concept analysis. *International Journal of Palliative Nursing, 13*(9), 451–460.

Kaut, K. P. (2002). Religions, spirituality, and existentialism near the end of life: Implications for assessment and application. *American Behavioral Scientist, 46*(2), 220–234. http://doi.org/10.1177/000276402236675.

Keall, R. M., Butow, P. N., Steinhauser, K. E., & Clayton, J. M. (2011). Discussing life story, forgiveness, heritage, and legacy with patients with life-limiting illnesses. *International Journal of Palliative Nursing, 17*(9), 454–461.

Kearney, M., & Mount, B. (2000). Spiritual care of the dying patient. In E. Chochinov, M. Harvey, & W. Breitbart (Eds.), *Handbook of psychiatry in palliative medicine* (pp. 357–373). Cary, NC: Oxford University Press.

Kellehear, A. (2000). Spirituality and palliative care: A model of needs. *Palliative Medicine, 14*, 149–155.

Kiely, B. E., Tattersall, M. H. N., & Stockler, M. R. (2010). Certain death in uncertain time: Informing hope by quantifying a best case scenario. *Journal of Clinical Oncology: Official Journal of the American Society of Clinical Oncology, 28*(16), 2802–2804. http://doi.org/10.1200/JCO.2009.27.3326.

King, M. B., & Koenig, H. G. (2009). Conceptualising spirituality for medical research and health service provision. *BMC Health Services Research, 9*, 116. http://doi.org/10.1186/1472-6963-9-116.

Kissane, D. W. (2012). The relief of existential suffering. *Archives of Internal Medicine, 172*(19), 1501–1505. http://doi.org/10.1001/archinternmed.2012.3633.

Lee, V. (2008). The existential plight of cancer: Meaning making as a concrete approach to the intangible search for meaning. *Supportive Care Cancer, 16*(7) 779–785. http://doi.org/10.1007/s00520-007-0396-7.

Lee, V., & Cohen, S. R. (2004). Clarifying "meaning" in the context of cancer research: A systematic literature review. *Palliative & Supportive Care, 2*(3), 291–303.

Lee, V., Cohen, S. R., Edgar, L., Laizner, A. M., & Gagnon, A. J. (2006). Meaning-making and psychological adjustment to cancer: Development of an intervention and pilot results. *Oncology Nursing Forum, 33*(2), 291–302. http://doi.org/10.1188/06.ONF.291-302.

Lee, V., & Loiselle, C. G. (2012). The salience of existential concerns across the cancer control continuum. *Palliative & Supportive Care, 10*(2), 123–133. http://doi.org/10.1017/S1478951511000745.

LeMay, K., & Wilson, K. G. (2008). Treatment of existential distress in life threatening illness: A review of manualized interventions. *Clinical Psychology Review, 28*(3), 472–493. http://doi.org/10.1016/j.cpr.2007.07.013.

Lethborg, C., Aranda, S., & Bloch, D. K. (2008). The role of meaning in advanced cancer—Integrating the constructs of assumptive world, sense of coherence and meaning-based coping. *Journal of Psychosocial Oncology, 24*(1), 37–41.

Lichtenthal, W. G., Nilsson, M., Zhang, B., Trice, E. D., Kissane, D. W., & Prigerson, H. G. (2009). Do rates of mental disorders and existential distress among advanced stage cancer patients increase as death approaches? *Psycho-Oncology, 61*(2), 50–61.

Lin, H., & Bauer-Wu, S. M. (2003). Psycho-spiritual well-being in patients with advanced cancer: An integrative review of the literature. *Journal of Advanced Nursing, 44*(1), 69–80.

Little, M., & Sayers, E.-J. (2004). While there's life . . . hope and the experience of cancer. *Social Science & Medicine (1982), 59*(6), 1329–1337. http://doi.org/10.1016/j.socscimed.2004.01.014.

Lo, B., Ruston, D., Kates, L. W., Arnold, R. M., Cohen, C. B., Faber-langendoen, K., . . . Sulmasy, D. P. (2002). Discussing religious and spiritual issues at the end of life. *JAMA, 287*, 749–754.

McClain, C. S., Rosenfeld, B., & Breitbart, W. (2003). Effect of spiritual well-being on end-of-life despair in terminally-ill cancer patients. *Lancet, 361*(9369), 1603–1607. http://doi.org/10.1016/S0140-6736(03)13310-7.

McClement, S. E., & Chochinov, H. M. (2008). Hope in advanced cancer patients. *European Journal of Cancer (Oxford, England: 1990), 44*(8), 1169–1174. http://doi.org/10.1016/j.ejca.2008.02.031.

McGrath, P. (2003a). Religiosity and the challenge of terminal illness. *Death Studies, 27*(June), 881–899. http://doi.org/10.1080/07481180390241840.

McGrath, P. (2003b). Spiritual pain: A comparison of findings from survivors and hospice patients. *American Journal of Hospice and Palliative Medicine, 20*(1), 23–33. http://doi.org/10.1177/104990910302000109.

Miller, D. K., Chibnall, J. T., Videen, S. D., & Duckro, P. N. (2005). Supportive-affective group experience for persons with life-threatening illness: Reducing spiritual, psychological, and death-related distress in dying patients. *Journal of Palliative Medicine, 8*(2), 333–343. http://doi.org/10.1089/jpm.2005.8.333.

Moadel, A., Morgan, C., Fatone, A., Grennan, J., Carter, J., Laruffa, G., . . . Dutcher, J. (1999). Seeking meaning and hope: Self-reported spiritual and existential needs among an ethnically-diverse cancer patient population. *Psycho-Oncology, 8*(5), 378–385. Retrieved from www.ncbi.nlm.nih.gov/pubmed/10559797.

Morita, T., Kawa, M., Honke, Y., Kohara, H., Maeyama, E., Kizawa, Y., . . . Uchitomi, Y. (2004). Existential concerns of terminally ill cancer patients receiving specialized palliative care in Japan. *Supportive Care in Cancer: Official Journal of the Multinational Association of Supportive Care in Cancer, 12*(2), 137–140. http://doi.org/10.1007/s00520-003-0561-6.

Mount, B. M. (2003). The existential moment. *Palliative & Supportive Care, 1*(1), 93–96.

Mount, B. M., Boston, P. H., & Cohen, S. R. (2007). Healing connections: On moving from suffering to a sense of well-being. *Journal of Pain and Symptom Management, 33*(4), 372–388. http://doi.org/10.1016/j.jpainsymman.2006.09.014.

Nelson, C. J., Rosenfeld, B., Breitbart, W., & Galietta, M. (2002). Spirituality, religion, and depression in the terminally ill. *Psychosomatics, 43*(3), 213–220. http://doi.org/10.1176/appi.psy.43.3.213.

Nuland, S. (1994). *How we die: Reflections on life's final chapter.* New York: Alfred A. Knopf, Inc./Vintage Books.

Park, C. L., & Folkman, S. (1997). Meaning in the context of stress and coping. *Review of General Psychology, 1*(2), 115–144.

Peteet, J. R., & Balboni, M. J. (2013). Spirituality and religion in oncology. *CA: A Cancer Journal for Clinicians, 63*(4), 280–289. http://doi.org/10.1002/caac.21187.

Peterman, A. H., Fitchett, G., Brady, M. J., Hernandez, L., Cella, D. (2002). Measuring spiritual well-being in people with cancer: The functional assessment of chronic illness therapy–spiritual well-being scale. *Annals of Behavioral Medicine, 24*(1), 49–58.

Peterman, A. H., Reeve, C. L., Winford, E. C., Cotton, S., Salsman, J. M., McQuellon, R., . . . Campbell, C. (2014). Measuring meaning and peace with the FACIT-Spiritual Well-Being Scale: Distinction without a difference? *Psychological Assessment, 26*(1), 127–137. http://doi.org/10.1037/a0034805

Phelps, A. C., Maciejewski, P. K., Nilsson, M., Balboni, T. A., Wright, A. A., Paulk, M. E., . . . Prigerson, H. G. (2009). Religious coping and use of intensive life-prolonging care in patients with advanced cancer. *JAMA: The Journal of the American Medical Association, 301*(11), 1140–1146.

Pickrel, J. (2007). "Tell me your story": Using life review in counseling the terminally Ill. *Death Studies, 13*(1989), 127–135.

Piderman, K. M., Johnson, M. E., Frost, M. H., Atherton, P. J., Satele, D. V., Clark, M. M., . . . Rummans, T. A. (2014). Spiritual quality of life in advanced cancer patients receiving radiation therapy. *Psycho-Oncology, 23*, 216–221.

Piderman, K. M., Kung, S., Jenkins, S. M., Euerle, T. T., Yoder, T. J., Kwete, G. M., & Lapid, M. I. (2015). Respecting the spiritual side of advanced cancer care: A systematic review. *Current Oncology Reports, 17*(2), 429. http://doi.org/10.1007/s11912-014-0429-6.

Post, S. G., Puchalski, C. M., & Larson, D. B. (2000). Physicians and patient spirituality: Professional boundaries, competency, and ethics. *Annals of Internal Medicine, 132*(7), 578–583. Retrieved from www.ncbi.nlm.nih.gov/pubmed/10744595.

Puchalski, C. M. (2001). The role of spirituality in health care. *Proceedings (Baylor University). Medical Center), 14*(4), 352–357. Retrieved from www.ncbi.nlm.nih.gov/pubmed/24041177.

Puchalski, C. M. (2002). Spirituality and end-of-life care: A time for listening and caring. *Journal of Palliative Medicine, 5*(2), 289–294. http://doi.org/10.1089/109662102753641287.

Puchalski, C. M. (2012). Spirituality in the cancer trajectory. *Annals of Oncology: Official Journal of the European Society for Medical Oncology/ESMO, 23*(Suppl. 3), iii49–iii55. http://doi.org/10.1093/annonc/mds088.

Puchalski, C. M., Ferrell, B., Virani, R., Otis-Green, S., Baird, P., Bull, J., . . . Sulmasy, D. (2009). Improving the quality of spiritual care as a dimension of palliative care: The report of the Consensus Conference. *Journal of Palliative Medicine, 12*(10), 885–904. http://doi.org/10.1089/jpm.2009.0142.

Puchalski, C. M., Lunsford, B., Harris, M. H., & Miller, R. T. (2006). Interdisciplinary spiritual care for seriously ill and dying patients: A collaborative model. *Cancer Journal (Sudbury, Mass.), 12*(5), 398–416. Retrieved from http://www.ncbi.nlm.nih.gov/pubmed/17034676.

Puchalski, C. M., & O'Donnell, E. (2005). Religious and spiritual beliefs in end of life care: How major religions view death and dying. *Techniques in Regional*

Anesthesia and Pain Management, 9(3), 114–121. http://doi.org/10.1053/j. trap.2005.06.003.

Puchalski, C. M., & Romer, A. L. (2000). Taking a spiritual history allows clinicians to understand patients more fully. *Journal of Palliative Medicine, 3*(1), 129–137. http://doi.org/10.1089/109662103322654839.

Pyszczynski, T., Greenberg, J., & Solomon, S. (1999). A dual-process model of defense against conscious and unconscious death-related thoughts: An extension of Terror Management Theory. *Psychological Review, 106*(4), 835–845.

Richardson, P. (2014). Spirituality, religion and palliative care. *Annals of Palliative Medicine, 3*(3), 150–159. http://doi.org/10.3978/j.issn.2224-5820.2014.07.05.

Robinson, S., Kissane, D. W., Brooker, J., & Burney, S. (2015). A systematic review of the demoralization syndrome in individuals with progressive disease and cancer: A decade of research. *Journal of Pain and Symptom Management, 49*(3), 595–610. http://doi.org/10.1016/j.jpainsymman.2014.07.008.

Rosenbaum, E., Garlan, R., Hirschberger, N., Siegel, A., Butler, L., & Spiegel, D. (2006). The Life Tape Project: Increasing family social support and symbolic immortality with a brief existential intervention for cancer patients and their families. *OMEGA—The Journal of Death and Dying, 53*(4), 321–339. http:// doi.org/10.2190/F143-5363-3442-5163.

Saunders, C. (2001). The evolution of palliative care. *Journal of the Royal Society of Medicine, 94*(9), 430–432. Retrieved from www.pubmedcentral.nih.gov/articler ender.fcgi?artid=1282179&tool=pmcentrez&rendertype=abstract.

Saunders, C., & Clark, D. (1999). "Total pain," disciplinary power and the body in the work of Cicely Saunders, 1958–1967. *Journal of Social Science and Medicine, 49*(6), 727–736.

Sharma, R. K., Astrow, A. B., Texeira, K., & Sulmasy, D. P. (2012). The spiritual needs assessment for patients (SNAP): Development and validation of a comprehensive instrument to assess unmet spiritual needs. *Journal of Pain and Symptom Management, 44*(1), 44–51. http://doi.org/10.1016/j.jpainsymman.2011.07.008.

Shuster, J. L., Breitbart, W., & Chochinov, H. M. (1999). Psychiatric aspects of excellent end-of-life care. *Psychosomatics, 40*(1), 1–4. http://doi.org/10.1016/S0033-3182(99)71265-X.

Sinclair, S., Bouchal, S. R., Chochinov, H., Hagen, N., & McClement, S. E. (2012). Spiritual care: How to do it. *BMJ Supportive & Palliative Care, 2*(4), 319–327. http://doi.org/10.1136/bmjspcare-2011-000191.

Steinhauser, K. E., Alexander, S. C., Byock, I. R., George, L. K., Olsen, M. K., & Tulsky, J. A. (2008). Do preparation and life completion discussions improve functioning and quality of life in seriously ill patients? Pilot randomized control trial. *Journal of Palliative Medicine, 11*(9), 1234–1240. http://doi.org/10.1089/jpm.2008.0078.

Steinhauser, K. E., Alexander, S. C., Byock, I. R., George, L. K., & Tulsky, J. A. (2009). Seriously ill patients' discussions of preparation and life completion: An intervention to assist with transition at the end of life. *Palliative & Supportive Care, 7*(4), 393–404. http://doi.org/10.1017/S147895150999040X.

Steinhauser, K. E., Christakis, N. A., Clipp, E. C., McNeilly, M., McIntyre, L., & Tulsky, J. A. (2000). Factors considered important at the end of life by patients, family, physicians, and other care providers. *JAMA: The Journal of the American Medical Association, 284*(19), 2476–2482. http://doi.org/10.1001/jama.284.19.2476.

Steinhauser, K. E., Clipp, E. C., McNeilly, M., Christakis, N. A., McIntyre, L. M., & Tulsky, J. A. (2000). In search of a good death: Observations of patients, families, and providers. *Annals of Internal Medicine, 132*(10), 825–832. Retrieved from www.ncbi.nlm.nih.gov/pubmed/10819707.

Steinhauser, K. E., Voils, C. I., Clipp, E. C., Bosworth, H. B., Christakis, N. A., Tulsky, J. A. (2006). "Are you at peace?" One item to probe spiritual concerns at the end of life. *Archives of Internal Medicine, 166*, 102–105.

Sulmasy, D. P. (2002). A biopsychosocial-spiritual model for the care of patients at the end of life. *The Gerontologist, 42*(Spec. No. III), 24–33. Retrieved from www.ncbi.nlm.nih.gov/pubmed/12415130.

Sulmasy, D. P. (2006). Spiritual issues in the care of dying patients. *JAMA: The Journal of the American Medical Association, 296*(11), 1385–1392.

SUPPORT Principal Investigators (1995). A controlled trial to improve care for seriously ill hospitalized patients, *JAMA, 274*(20), 1591–1598.

Surbone, A., & Baider, L. (2010). The spiritual dimension of cancer care. *Critical Reviews in Oncology/Hematology, 73*(3), 228–235. http://doi.org/10.1016/j.critrevonc.2009.03.011.

Tarakeshwar, N., Vanderwerker, L. C., Paulk, E., Pearce, M. J., Kasl, S. V., & Prigerson, H. G. (2006). Religious coping is associated with the quality of life of patients with advanced cancer. *Journal of Palliative Medicine, 9*(3), 646–657. http://doi.org/10.1089/jpm.2006.9.646.

Vachon, M., Fillion, L., & Achille, M. (2009). A conceptual analysis of spirituality at the end of life. *Journal of Palliative Medicine, 12*(1), 53–59. http://doi.org/10.1089/jpm.2008.0189.

Vallurupalli, M., Lauderdale, K., Balboni, M. J., Phelps, A. C., Block, S. D., Kachnic, G.A.K., VanderWeele, L. A., Balboni, T. A. (2012). The role of spirituality and religious coping in the quality of life of patients with advanced cancer receiving palliative radiation therapy. *Journal of Supportive Oncology, 10*(2), 81–87. http://doi.org/10.1016/j.suponc.2011.09.003.The

Vig, E. K., & Pearlman, R. A. (2003). Quality of life while dying: A qualitative study of terminally ill older men. *Journal of the American Geriatrics Society, 51*, 1595–1601.

Walter, T. (1997). The ideology and organization of spiritual care: Three approaches. *Palliative Medicine, 11*, 21–30.

Walter, T. (2002). Spirituality in palliative care: opportunity or burden? *Palliative Medicine, 16*, 133–39. http://doi.org/10.1191/0269216302pm516oa.

Weisman, A. D. (1972). *On dying and denying.* New York: Behavioral Publications, Inc.

Weisman, A. D., & Worden, J. W. (1976–77). The existential plight in cancer: Significance of the first 100 days. *International Journal of Psychiatry in Medicine, 7*(1), 1–15.

Whitford, H. S., & Olver, I. N. (2012). The multidimensionality of spiritual wellbeing: Peace, meaning, and faith and their association with quality of life and coping in oncology. *Psycho-Oncology, 21*, 602–610.

Winkelman, W. D., Lauderdale, K., Balboni, M. J., Phelps, A. C., Peteet, J. R., Block, S. D., . . . Balboni, T. A. (2011). The relationship of spiritual concerns to the quality of life of advanced cancer patients: Preliminary findings. *Journal of Palliative Medicine, 14*(9), 1022–1028. http://doi.org/10.1089/jpm.2010.0536.

Yang, W., Staps, T., & Hijmans, E. (2010). Existential crisis and the awareness of dying: The role of meaning and spirituality. *OMEGA—Journal of Death and Dying, 61*(1), 53–69. http://doi.org/10.2190/OM.61.1.c.

7 Psychotherapeutic Interventions in End-of-life Care

> . . . the idea of death, the fear of it, haunts the human animal like nothing else; it is a mainspring of human activity—activity designed largely to avoid the fatality of death, to overcome it by denying that it is in some way the final destiny for man.
>
> (Becker, 1973, p. ix)

The diagnosis of a life-threatening illness presents a challenge to an individual's assumptive world, a struggle to make sense of the illness. Even if the diagnosis was expected or feared, the patient may feel an existential sense of abandonment, that one's god has left him/her to face the crisis alone. Patients struggle to decide whether their life as lived has a sense of meaning and purpose and to seek forgiveness for unaccomplished tasks or for hurtful acts committed. Individuals seek to die an appropriate death and to find hope beyond the grave; they wish to be remembered as life continues with the hope that they will live on in the genes of their family members and in the creations and legacies they leave (Chochinov, 2002; Breitbart, 2001).

Psychotherapeutic interventions have been formulated to assist patients in grappling with these issues, particularly those individuals in palliative care with end stage cancer or other life-limiting diseases. These important interventions are showing great success at impacting patient's existential well-being and other psychological issues such as depression (Whitford & Olver, 2012). These interventions view meaning as a general life orientation, as personal significance, as causality, as a coping mechanism, and as an outcome. The construct of meaning is critically important to the psychosocial adjustment to terminal illness. Psychosocial interventions often include components of the meaning-making process (Nissim et al., 2012; Lo et al., 2014), and multi-modal supportive care interventions, including supportive-expressive, cognitive-behavioral, couples-based (McLean et al., 2013), or psychoeducational techniques (see Holland et al., 2009).

Supportive psychotherapy is the mainstay used to bolster adaptive coping strategies or minimize maladaptive ones. Insight-oriented therapies have had limited use with dying patients. Interpersonal therapy has been used with HIV/AIDS patients to help reframe depression caused by their disease, but has not been used with dying patients because of its long duration. Group supportive psychotherapy, including self-help groups, brings together patients with similar diseases to share information. While many interventions have been attempted and/or written about in the literature, this section reviews only those therapies that have been amply tested and found to be valid to promote quality of life and a good death in patients nearing death.

Breitbart's Meaning-Centered Group Therapy (MCGT), with its basis in Logotherapy, and Chochinov's Dignity Therapy, are interventions used with dying patients who remain sufficiently robust to participate in a two-month intervention. Existential supportive/expressive group psychotherapy was developed by Yalom and Spiegel, and has been used by Virginia Lee in MMi interventions, to work with patients suffering from breast cancer on ways to deal with their terminal illness. Kissane et al.'s (2004, 2007) supportive-expressive group therapy (SEGT) is rooted in the principles of existential psychotherapy and includes instruction on coping skills and effective communication with healthcare providers. Cognitive behavioral therapy (CBT) is used in cancer populations to correct cognitive distortions, establish coping strategies, and mobilize inner resources; Greer et al. (2010, 2012) adapted the basic theories of CBT into a novel, shorter form to benefit patients at the end of life (Chochinov et al., 2004, pp. 136–7).

7.1 LOGOTHERAPY

> . . . logotherapy, in comparison with psychoanalysis, is a method less *retrospective* and less *introspective*. Logotherapy focuses rather on the future, that is to say, on the meanings to be fulfilled by the patient in his future. (Logotherapy indeed is a meaning centered psychotherapy.)
>
> (Frankl, 1984, p. 120)

Viktor E. Frankl, number 119104, experienced concentration camps as an ordinary prisoner. In order to cope with the inhumane conditions, the prisoner relied on the intensity of his inner life as a way to take refuge from "the desolation and the spiritual poverty" of his existence (Frankl, 1984, pp. 58–9). Frankl experienced the beauty of art and of nature as his inner life intensified still further. Even though suffering was omnipresent, he found it possible to develop a sense of humor and to experience joy. Frankl specified that these options were personal, purposeful choices, not the result of camp influences alone: prisoners had the choice of deciding what would become of them, emotionally and mentally, retaining human dignity even in a concentration camp: "The way in which a man accepts his fate and all the suffering it entails, the way in which he takes up his cross, gives him ample opportunity—even under the most difficult circumstances—to add a deeper meaning to his life" (Frankl, 1984, p. 88).

Logotherapy has also been termed The Third Viennese School of Psychotherapy. Frankl believed that the primary motivational force in man was to find meaning in one's life. Logotherapy is a meaning-centered psychotherapy in which the patient is "confronted with and reoriented toward the meaning of his life" (Frankl, 1984, p. 120). Logotherapy involves a focus on the meaning of human existence and that "this striving to find a meaning in one's life is the primary motivational force in man" (p. 121). Frankl's view of meaning is borne out in the central role of the meaning-making function in various related psychotherapeutic approaches, and their common premise that "we as humans have a need to make sense of the world" (Hack et al., 2010, p. 721). Logotherapy is unlike traditional psychotherapies that focus on psychopathology and psychological symptoms, to "specifically address a patient's strengths and his or her personal search for meaning and purpose in life" (Southwick et al., 2006, p. 163). The loss of meaning and purpose experienced by some terminally ill individuals has pronounced effects on psychosocial functioning and these may be heightened by meaning-based psychotherapies.

Frankl noted three inevitable existential problems: suffering, death, and guilt (existential guilt about the fact that one never lives up to one's potential). Some of Frankl's basic concepts concern:

1. Meaning of life—life has meaning and never ceases to have meaning even up to the last moment of life: meaning may change in this context but it never ceases to exist (1984, p. 131).
2. Will to meaning—the desire to find meaning in human existence is a primary instinct and basic motivation for human behavior (1984, p. 121).
3. Freedom of will—we have the freedom to find meaning in existence and to choose our attitude to suffering.

Other of Frankl's basic ideas include the concept that "life is a gift and that we have a responsibility to live life to the fullest; meaning occurs in the historical context of an individual, his family, his people, humankind" (Breitbart, 2001, p. 9).

The meaning of life is different for each of us, always changes but never ceases to be. According to Logotherapy, one can find the meaning of life in three different ways: (1) by creating a work or doing a deed; (2) by experiencing something or encountering someone; and (3) by the attitude we take to unavoidable suffering (Frankl, 1984, p. 133). Frankl focused on suffering as an opportunity to find meaning and thereby "to transform a personal tragedy into a triumph" (p. 135), an opportunity for a person to rise above a fate he cannot change and grow beyond it. Thereby, the suffering one has gone through has been done with courage and dignity, so that

Frankl cautioned against the young pitying the old: "instead of possibilities in the future, they have realities in the past—the potentialities they have actualized, the meanings they have fulfilled, the values they have realized" (p. 175), which nobody can remove from the past.

A comprehensive intervention to address the *emotional and spiritual distress* of patients with advanced life-limiting illness, called OUTLOOK, was developed in 2009 by Steinhauser et al. The intervention is similar to Frankl's Logotherapy and shares goals with Chochinov's Dignity Therapy, but is not a psychotherapeutic intervention. The intervention was a three-day protocol designed to be brief, transportable, and manualized, which "guides participants through discussions of elements of end-of-life preparation and completion" (Steinhauser et al., 2009, p. 394). The first session focused on three aspects of the patient's life story: a description telling about their lives, cherished times to evoke "personal values and strengths", and personal accomplishments (p. 397). The second interview asked patients to reflect on what they might have done differently and on life regrets, forgiveness, and whether they were at peace. The section on what patients thought they might have done differently revealed that while there were things patients may have done differently, they would not have changed everything they did. The third interview regarded heritage and legacy "that focused on life lessons learned, lessons to share with loved ones and other generations, and issues of personal legacy" (p. 399) that often tied back to the elements of the first two interviews.

A patient's role is as a passive recipient of care (Steinhauser et al., 2009, p. 401) filled with suffering due to the prospect of a truncated future. Despite being surrounded by loved ones and friends, patients experience existential loneliness that is compounded by "a conspiracy of silence in which both the ill person and close relatives and friends avoid discussing their concerns about the gravity of the illness" (p. 401). Such avoidant behavior threatens the patient's sense of being intact. The OUTLOOK intervention sought to allow patients to reconnect with the intact persons they were prior to their illness.

7.2 MEANING-CENTERED PSYCHOTHERAPY

> Even under normal conditions, a strong meaning orientation is a life-prolonging, if not a life-preserving agent.
>
> (Frankl, 1966, p. 103)

Dr. William Breitbart and his research group at Memorial Sloan Kettering Cancer Center were interested in the emerging importance of spiritual well-being and, especially, the role of meaning "in moderating depression, hopelessness and desire for death in terminally ill cancer and AIDS patients" (Breitbart, 2001, p. 8). They developed a novel, non-pharmacologic intervention to combat such issues in patients with advanced cancer at the end of life. Breitbart et al. (Breitbart, 2001; Breitbart & Heller, 2003) saw a way of adapting Frankl's Logotherapy and its focus on spirituality and meaning for psychotherapeutic work with patients at the end of life. Many such patients seek help in understanding cancer and impending death in the context of their lives, as well as ways of sustaining meaning and hope (Breitbart et al., 2004).

The chosen format of the intervention initially was a group intervention. The team posited that the group model may offer benefits not available in individual settings, such as: a sense of universality; sharing a common experience and identity; a feeling of helping oneself by helping others; hopefulness fostered by seeing how others have coped successfully; and a sense of belonging to a larger group (self-*transcendence*, meaning, common purpose).

The goal of this psychotherapeutic intervention, Meaning-Centered Group Psychotherapy (MCGP), is to help men and women with advanced cancer focus on "what has been, and can still be, meaningful in their lives given their circumstances, and to further develop their ability to reframe their experience from that of dying to that of living despite the threat of dying" (Greenstein & Breitbart, 2000, p. 491). The team manualized a novel eight-week intervention, consisting of 1 to 1.5 hours each week that utilizes a mixture of didactics, discussion, and experiential exercises focused around particular themes related to meaning and advanced cancer. The session themes include:

> Session 1: Concepts of meaning and sources of meaning
> Session 2: Cancer and meaning
> Session 3: Meaning and historical context of life
> Session 4: Storytelling, life project
> Session 5: Limitations and finiteness of life
> Session 6: Responsibility, creativity, deeds
> Session 7: Experience, nature, art, humor
> Session 8: Termination, goodbyes, hopes for the future

Patients were assigned reading and homework relating to each week's theme that are discussed in session. The focus of the intervention is on finding peace and meaning in the face of a limited prognosis.

The ultimate goal of this intervention is the effective use of coping in order to enhance patients' sense of meaning and purpose, so that each group member makes the most of his or her time, no matter how limited it may be. It is up to each member to use the group to find sources of meaning in his or her life, so that they are active participants in the process. Participants must be willing to help create meaning, for themselves as well as for the other members, "since the concept of the intervention is as a creative, individual, and active process" (Breitbart et al., 2004, p. 371).

Breitbart et al. (2010) performed a study of MCGP. Few interventions to date had been developed for the population of elderly terminal cancer patients and those few that had did not have as their primary outcomes the effects of spirituality and well-being. The study demonstrated significantly greater benefits from spiritual well-being and meaning for the MCGP participants than those from the supportive group psychotherapy (SGP) control group. Also, the treatment benefits remained and even grew, as shown at a two-month post-test, while participants in the SGP failed to show any such improvement. Patients in the MCGP experienced a lessening of psychological distress and a small lowering of feelings of hopelessness, anxiety, and desire for death.

The 2010 trial of MCGP resulted in substantial attrition, such that Breitbart et al. (2010, 2015) saw the need of further studies in which group therapy was replaced by individual therapy (IMGT). The team performed a randomized pilot study on the new version in 2012. The comparison group likewise had to be an individual intervention, so Therapeutic Massage (TM) was chosen, as it had been shown beneficial, as opposed to standard care, in relieving anxiety, mood disturbance, and physical symptom distress. The IMCP was a manualized psychotherapeutic intervention of seven weeks' duration, each session lasting for one hour, designed for patients with advanced cancer to enhance or sustain a sense of meaning, peace, and purpose to a life being diminished by the progression of illness. The individual format was "intended to increase the flexibility of treatment implementation because scheduling or illness-related problems often hinder attendance in a group intervention, particularly with individuals who have advanced cancer" (Breitbart et al., 2012, p. 1306). All other program facilitation was the same as the prior MCGP. The results of the IMCP replicated and extended those of the MCGP, but with lower attrition rates. However, IMCP demonstrated a lack of improvement at the two-month follow-up, a difference from the MCGP.

7.3 DIGNITY THERAPY

> Patients provided countless examples of times when the behaviours of family, friends, and health providers served to enhance or diminish their dignity. Patients also shared descriptions about those things that gave their life meaning . . . and named the essential life activities, attitudes, and self-philosophies that fostered their feelings of personal dignity. For many patients, . . . life without dignity was described as a life no longer worthy of living. . . . Thus, the concept of dignity and the dignity model may offer a way of understanding how patients navigate the wish to go on living.
>
> (Chochinov et al., 2002, p. 441)

Dignity Therapy is a brief, individualized psychotherapeutic intervention designed to address psychosocial and existential distress among terminally ill patients (Chochinov et al., 2005a; McClement et al., 2004). Such distress is associated with the concepts of suffering and lack of meaning that threaten the intactness of a dying person. Dignity Therapy engages terminal patients in a brief, individualized intervention designed to foster a sense of meaning and purpose, in order to reduce suffering.

The dignity model of palliative care, a review of which is presented here, provides the framework for this novel intervention and informs its content and therapeutic tone: to decrease suffering, enhance quality of life, and bolster a sense of meaning, purpose, and dignity. Employing Dignity Therapy, dying patients are offered the opportunity to address those issues that matter most to them and to address things they would most want remembered as death draws near (Chochinov et al., 2005a, p. 5521).

The Model of Dignity in the Terminally Ill

> Unlike most other symptom-focused interventions, the beneficial effects of dignity therapy reside in being able to bolster a sense of meaning and purpose while reinforcing a continued sense of worth within a framework that is supportive, nurturing, and accessible, even for those proximate to death.
>
> (Chochinov et al., 2005a, p. 5524)

Items contained in a qualitative 2006 study of the Dignity Model provided a broad and inclusive range of issues and concerns that influence a dying patient's sense of dignity. The study items most highly endorsed included not feeling supported by your community, not feeling worthwhile or valued, not being able to manage bodily functions, not feeling you have made a meaningful or lasting contribution, not feeling you have control over your life, feeling a burden to others, and not being treated with respect or understanding; the last two items were the most highly endorsed dignity-related concerns (Chochinov et al., 2006, p. 670; Chochinov, 2007; Chochinov et al., 2007).

Maintaining dignity often was found to be highly dependent on the tone of care, the overall sensitivity of the support network within which care is delivered, termed illness related issues; for others, dignity was undermined by the illness experience itself, or illness-related issues, as experienced proportionately to the degree of symptom distress and physical limitations or losses imposed by the encroaching cancer; and for some patients, maintaining a sense of dignity was dependent upon personal approaches or outlooks determined by long-standing personality characteristics, attitudes, or philosophies, called the dignity conserving repertoire (Chochinov, Hack, Hassard, et al., 2002, p. 2029; Chochinov, 2002).

Dignity-Conserving Care: The Dignity Therapy Protocol

Dignity-conserving care is "care that confers honour, and recognises the deservedness of respect and esteem of every individual—despite their dependency, infirmity, and fragility" (Chochinov, Hack, Hassard, et al., 2002, p. 2029). The themes of the Dignity Therapy protocol are based in the categories and themes of the dignity model developed and piloted by Chochinov's team. The protocol provides an intervention that is a brief, manualized psychotherapy that can be accomplished at the patient's bedside; it is designed to benefit patients who have the cognitive ability to participate. All protocol questions afford patients a means of speaking to the issues that might reinforce their personhood, meaning, self-worth, and purpose in order to decrease distress or bolster quality of life. Most of the dignity model sub-themes of generativity, continuity of self, maintaining pride and hope, role preservation, burden to others, and aftermath concerns provide patients the means to create a legacy document that addresses aspects of life the patient feels proudest of, are most meaningful, and reflect the personal history the patient would most want remembered (Chochinov et al., 2005a; Fitchett et al., 2015). Dignity Therapy sessions are taped, transcribed, and edited, and the transcripts quickly returned to the patient. The transcripts are intended to be left for family or loved ones and form "part of a personal legacy that the patient will have helped shape and create" (Chochinov et al., 2004, p. 140; McClement et al., 2004).

The feasibility study (Chochinov et al., 2005a) began with patients being asked to take baseline psychometrics and then to participate in a 30- or 60-minute audiotaped session focused on the things that mattered to them most, and questions that were supplied to patients before the audiotaping. The patients' audiotaped transcripts were reshaped and read to the patients for their comments and changes. At the conclusion of the intervention, quantitative measures were re-administered and a Dignity Therapy survey disseminated, allowing the patients to reflect on their experience.

Post-intervention measures of suffering and of depressed mood revealed significant improvement while the post-intervention measures of dignity approached significance. Patients who reported higher levels of psychosocial despair benefitted from Dignity Therapy in particular. Finding the intervention helpful was significantly correlated with finding life more meaningful (Chochinov et al., 2005a). Likewise, the team used questionnaires to follow up with family members of deceased patients who had participated in Dignity Therapy. Their endorsement of Dignity Therapy was completely positive and revealed the intervention also to be beneficial to bereaved family members (McClement et al., 2007; van Gennip et al., 2013). These results were validated by a Chinese study (Ho et al., 2013), with the exception of noting the need to develop more culturally sensitive and family-oriented interventions for reducing the existential pain of dying among Chinese patients in Hong Kong. A 2011 study by Montross et al. described the practicalities of implementing Dignity Therapy in a community-based hospice setting.

The Patient Dignity Inventory (PDI), a novel 25-item psychometric screening instrument, was designed to measure and identify multiple sources of distress (physical, functional, psychosocial, existential, and spiritual) commonly seen in terminally ill patients. The PDI was developed to afford new opportunities in examining and better understanding the landscape of dignity-related distress among patients nearing death. The instrument was also designed to help inform psychosocial clinicians working with these patients and its validity and reliability have been studied within the context of palliative care and in clinical settings. The PDI afforded a better grasp of the nature of distress in the terminally ill (Chochinov et al., 2009), including insight regarding those who are most at risk and can pave the way toward more effective, dignity conserving end-of-life care and a good death (Chochinov et al., 2008, 2009, 2011).

A 2011 study of a multi-site randomized controlled trial, with patients assigned to Dignity Therapy, Client Centered Care (focused on non-generativity, here and now issues), or Standard Palliative Care arms, was conducted to determine if Dignity Therapy was able to mitigate distress and/or bolster end-of-life experience for patients nearing death. Whereas ample evidence was provided by the study that Dignity Therapy was a viable clinical intervention for terminal patients, the study did not prove its ability to alleviate distress, such as depression, desire for death or for suicide. A post-study survey, revealed that patients who received Dignity Therapy were significantly more likely to report benefits, "in terms of finding it helpful, improving their quality of life, their sense of dignity; changing how their family might see or appreciate them, and deeming it helpful to their family, compared to the other study arms" (Chochinov et al., 2011, p. 759).

Perceived lack of caring and of good communication skills of doctors towards patients have been a standard complaint voiced by patients and their families since before the SUPPORT studies. Physician researchers, educators, and clinicians, in various specialties, have researched the question. Chochinov et al. (2014) formulated and presented a very simple, direct and to-the-point intervention that solved the problem: to ask the patients and/ or families what they want the clinicians to know about them. Called the Patient Dignity Question (PDQ), the written answer to the PDQ serves to acknowledge the personhood of the patient. With consent to place the document in the patient chart, the information reflects what the patient/family values and wishes everyone who is taking care of them to know. The knowledge of what matters to the patients and who they are as persons facilitates medical decision making and improves diagnostic accuracy and patient safety. Answering this simple question gives patients a voice in expressing their needs and preferences, thereby bringing them closer to the reality of meaning and dignity in death (Proulx, 2004). The PDQ does not replace communication among doctors and patients, but offers an effective way to open the door to further information about personhood.

The aim of a 2010 study by Hack et al. was to capture the voices of the dying from randomly drawn Dignity Therapy transcripts. These revealed that, as death draws near, a natural process of reflection, framing a thoughtful remembrance of the meaningful experiences of a life lived, takes place (Hack et al., 2010, p. 716). The transcripts showed that dying patients commonly use Dignity Therapy to affirm significant others, and to express wishes and gratitude to others.

Chochinov et al. (2005a) made the point that few non-pharmacological interventions are specifically designed to lessen the suffering or existential distress that often accompanies patients at the end of life. He pointed out that the rationale of most of these interventions is to make the sufferer less aware of "his or her suffering, and are the equivalent of emotional analgesia without necessarily addressing the source or cause of the underlying psychic pain" (Chochinov et al., 2005a, p. 5524). Chochinov's Dignity Therapy was therefore developed to treat the source of the underlying psychic pain. Unlike most other symptom-focused interventions, the beneficial effects of Dignity Therapy reside in being able to bolster a sense of meaning and purpose while reinforcing a continued sense of worth that is supportive, nurturing, and accessible even for those proximate to death (Chochinov et al., 2005a).

Multiple studies of Dignity Therapy, qualitative studies of Dignity Therapy, and case reports on the use of Dignity Therapy, have been conducted that describe widespread acceptability and high satisfaction among patients/ families who experienced it (Fitchett et al., 2015, pp. 4–8). While challenges to the model exist, Fitchett et al.'s literature review found "robust evidence for DT's overwhelming acceptability, rare for any medical intervention, especially in psycho-social-spiritual care" (p. 10).

7.4 COGNITIVE-BEHAVIORAL THERAPY (CBT)

> Psychiatric disorders such as depression, anxiety and delirium occur in a significant percentage of cancer patients, particularly as disease advances and as cancer treatments become more aggressive.
>
> (Breitbart, 1995, p. 45)

Patients with advanced cancer experience incapacitating anxiety symptoms that interfere with their quality of life and produce poor medical outcomes. CBT is an empirically validated psychotherapeutic treatment of choice in clinical trials; however, clinical trials of CBT exclude comorbidities in general and cancer in particular. CBT is used to treat anxiety disorders featuring unrealistic fears and worries in healthy populations, whereas advanced cancer symptoms present with realistic fears (Greer et al., 2010; Greer et al., 2012).

Researchers found a high incidence of patients with anxiety disorders comorbid with advanced cancer. Such elevated anxiety levels in persons with advanced cancer have been associated with symptoms such as dyspnea, fatigue, nausea, and pain, as well as a poor quality of life. Persons with an anxiety disorder premorbid to a cancer diagnosis face an exacerbation of those anxiety symptoms in the face of the realities of a life-threatening disease. Others without an anxiety disorder facing such a diagnosis will experience growing anxiety symptoms during the major transitions of the disease state (Greer et al., 2010; Greer et al., 2012).

Existing studies of psychosocial interventions for anxiety comorbid with cancer did not sufficiently employ CBT techniques in patients with later stage cancer. Also, this population faced significantly realistic anxiety symptoms that existing CBT interventions did not address. Therefore, Greer and colleagues saw the necessity of tailoring a cognitive-based intervention to benefit late stage cancer patients with complex medical symptoms and progressive loss of functioning. Specifically, the team made concerted efforts to provide easy access to psychotherapy sessions and also "adapted our CBT approach to incorporate skills for managing realistic, cancer-related worries and progressive disability" (Greer et al., 2012, p. 1338).

The intervention consisted of six or seven weekly sessions with four modules of the following topics: (1) one session on education about anxiety and on goal setting; (2) one session on relaxation training; (3) three sessions on coping with cancer fears; and (4) one or two sessions on activity planning and pacing. Each module included homework assignments and skills practice (Greer et al., 2010; Greer et al., 2012). Two arms of the study comprised the CBT arm and the waitlist control arm, whose participants could crossover to the CBT arm after the eight-week posttest assessment of the CBT group was completed (Greer et al., 2012).

The results of this pilot feasibility and randomized controlled trial of brief CBT comorbid with terminal cancer revealed significant beneficial effects of the therapy in reducing anxiety symptoms. Compared to the waitlist control group, the team "observed marginally significant improvements in emotional and functional well-being in those assigned to CBT" (Greer et al., 2012, p. 1344), in spite of declines in physical well-being over time.

7.5 EXISTENTIAL THERAPIES

[Existential psychotherapy] addresses the inner conflict and anxiety born out of our awareness of the vulnerability we experience as a product of the existential givens that frame our lives. These givens, our ultimate concerns, include **death** (existential obliteration), **freedom** (the absence of external structure), **isolation** (the final unbridgeable gap separating self from all else), and the **question of meaning** (the dilemma of meaning seeking creatures who recognize the possibility of the cosmos without meaning).

(Kearney & Mount, 2000, p. 359; bold in source)

When people are confronted with issues about their mortality, such as being presented with a diagnosis of cancer, an existential crisis may ensue.

Individuals may then need to learn to cope with loss of meaning and empowerment, which can compromise quality of life. Existential therapies are psychological interventions that are informed, to a significant extent, by the teachings of existential philosophers such as Heidegger, Sartre, Buber, Tillich, Kierkegaard, and Nietzsche. These therapies are a group of psychological interventions that explicitly address questions about existence based on one or more existential philosophical assumptions. The existential dimension is an integral part of human experience, including but not limited to spiritual and religious aspects, which attempts to address questions about human existence and all that is connected to one's reason for being.

Living with a terminal illness amplifies existential concerns of death, meaning, freedom, and isolation, such that one aim of the existential-based interventions is to give patients an opportunity to discuss these concerns. The treatment strategy involves facilitating discussion of issues that are uppermost in patients' minds rather than imposing on the group the topics to be discussed. Investigation of existential therapies, such as supportive-expressive group psychotherapy, works by directly challenging patients' tendencies to withdraw and avoid the implications of their condition (Classen et al., 2001).

Cognitive-Existential Group Therapy (CEGT)

Kissane initiated work on CEGT to deal with issues that specifically arise in the newly diagnosed patient, as opposed to his subsequent work with advanced disease states. His group devised and piloted an approach that incorporated existential and cognitive dimensions (Kissane et al., 2003) that emphasized education, cognitive reappraisal, and promotion of enhanced coping pertinent to those with early stage cancers, in conjunction with existentially oriented and supportive-expressive strategies, the latter two originally used in the advanced cancer setting. A group model was favored in view of its potential to promote a supportive environment and because of its cost effectiveness. The randomized, controlled trial of CEGT with women with early stage breast cancer receiving adjuvant chemotherapy ran into methodological problems but showed promise. Kissane's treatment team preferred the use of a cognitively oriented model in early stage cancer with the goals of preparing for survivorship and living with uncertainty and fear of recurrence.

Supportive-Existential Group Therapy (SEGT)

Kissane et al. (2004) reported on a randomized control trial (RCT) of SEGT for women with advanced breast cancer. He specified the goals of the RCT as "building bonds, expressing emotions, 'detoxifying' death and dying, redefining life's priorities, fortifying families and friends, enhancing doctor–patient relationships and improving coping" (p. 756), thus consolidating social support, and promoting collaborative patient–clinician communication. Therapists encourage group members to exchange telephone numbers and meet for refreshments after a session in order to promote regular exchange of medical information and personal happenings to counter existential aloneness. Members are guided to face the inherent presence of existential ambivalence: happiness and joy in life versus death and acceptance of mortality. SEGT has "clearly demonstrated improvement of quality of life and optimises adaptive adjustment and creative living during what is potentially one of life's most challenging transitions" (Kissane et al., 2004, p. 766).

Kissane et al. (2007) performed an RCT on SEGT to investigate survival and psychosocial outcomes in women with advanced metastatic breast cancer. Adding SEGT to standard oncology care in this population did not influence survival, but psychosocial outcomes improved. This RCT demonstrated that SEGT both treats and prevents depression, providing "another reason for group therapy to be seriously considered as an appropriate model of support for patients with advanced cancer" (p. 284).

Supportive psychosocial interventions to improve end-of-life care and to promote a good death have established a strong bedrock in psychotherapeutic techniques that began to be developed in the late 20 century. The concepts of dignity, meaning, and spiritual coping translated into beneficial techniques that bolster end-of-life care. Clinical trials of Dignity Therapy and Meaning-Centered Group Therapy have validated their high potential to foster good outcomes to benefit people approaching death.

CITATIONS: CHAPTER 7

Becker, E. (1973). *The denial of death*. New York: The Free Press/A Division of Macmillan Publishing.

Breitbart, W. (1995). Identifying patients at risk for, and treatment of major psychiatric complications of cancer. *Supportive Care in Cancer, 3*(1), 45–60.

Breitbart, W. (2001). Spirituality and meaning in supportive care: Spirituality- and meaning-centered group psychotherapy interventions in advanced cancer. *Supportive Care in Cancer: Official Journal of the Multinational Association of Supportive Care in Cancer, 10*(4), 1–15. http://doi.org/10.1007/s005200100289.

Breitbart, W., Bruera, E., Chochinov, H., & Lynch, M. (1995). Neuropsychiatric syndromes and psychological symptoms in patients with advanced cancer. *Journal of Pain and Symptom Management, 10*(2), 131–141. Retrieved from www.ncbi.nlm.nih.gov/pubmed/7730685.

Breitbart, W., Gibson, C., Poppito, S.R., & Berg, A. (2004). Psychotherapeutic interventions at the end of life: A focus on meaning and spirituality. *Canadian Journal of Psychiatry, 49*(6), 366–373.

Breitbart, W., & Heller, K.S. (2003). Reframing hope: Meaning-centered care for patients near the end of life. *Journal of Palliative Medicine, 6*(6), 979–988.

Breitbart, W., Poppito, S., Rosenfeld, B., Vickers, A.J., Li, Y., Abbey, J., . . . Cassileth, B.R. (2012). Pilot randomized controlled trial of individual meaning-centered psychotherapy for patients with advanced cancer. *Journal of Clinical Oncology, 30*(12), 1304–1309. http://doi.org/10.1200/JCO.2011.36.2517.

Breitbart, W., Rosenfeld, B., Gibson, C., Pessin, H., Poppito, S., Nelson, C., . . . Olden, M. (2010). Meaning-centered group psychotherapy for patients with advanced cancer: A pilot randomized controlled trial. *Psycho-Oncology, 19*(1), 21–28. http://doi.org/10.1002/pon.1556.

Breitbart, W., Rosenfeld, B., Pessin, H., Applebaum, A., Kulikowski, J., & Lichtenthal, W. G. (2015). Meaning-centered group psychotherapy: An effective intervention for improving psychological well-being in patients with advanced cancer. *Journal of Clinical Oncology: Official Journal of the American Society of Clinical Oncology, 33*(7), 749–754. http://doi.org/10.1200/JCO.2014.57.2198.

Chochinov, H. M. (2002). Dignity-conserving care—A new model for palliative care: Helping the patient feel valued. *JAMA: The Journal of the American Medical Association, 287*(17), 2253–2260. Retrieved from www.ncbi.nlm.nih.gov/pubmed/11980525.

Chochinov, H. M. (2007). Dignity and the essence of medicine: The A, B, C, and D of dignity conserving care. *BMJ (Clinical Research Ed.), 335*(7612), 184–187. http://doi.org/10.1136/bmj.39244.650926.47.

Chochinov, H. M. (2011). Death, time and the theory of relativity. *Journal of Pain and Symptom Management, 42*(3), 460–463. http://doi.org/10.1016/j.jpainsymman.2010.12.001.

Chochinov, H. M., Hack, T., Hassard, T., Kristjanson, L. J., McClement, S. E., & Harlos, M. (2002). Dignity in the terminally ill: A cross-sectional, cohort study. *Lancet, 360*(9350), 2026–2030. http://doi.org/10.1016/S0140-6736(02)12022-8.

Chochinov, H. M., Hack, T., Hassard, T., Kristjanson, L. J., McClement, S. E., & Harlos, M. (2004). Dignity and psychotherapeutic considerations in end-of-life care. *Journal of Palliative Care, 20*(3), 134–142.

Chochinov, H. M., Hack, T., Hassard, T., Kristjanson, L. J., McClement, S. E., & Harlos, M. (2005a). Dignity therapy: A novel psychotherapeutic intervention for patients near the end of life. *Journal of Clinical Oncology: Official Journal of the American Society of Clinical Oncology, 23*(24), 5520–5525. http://doi.org/10.1200/JCO.2005.08.391.

Chochinov, H. M., Hack, T., Hassard, T., Kristjanson, L. J., McClement, S. E., & Harlos, M. (2005b). Understanding the will to live in patients nearing death. *Psychosomatics, 46*, 7–10.

Chochinov, H. M., Hack, T., McClement, S. E., Kristjanson, L., & Harlos, M. (2002). Dignity in the terminally ill: A developing empirical model. *Social Science & Medicine (1982), 54*(3), 433–443. Retrieved from www.ncbi.nlm.nih.gov/pubmed/11824919.

Chochinov, H. M., Hassard, T., McClement, S. E., Hack, T., Kristjanson, L. J., Harlos, M., . . . Murray, A. (2008). The patient dignity inventory: A novel way of measuring dignity-related distress in palliative care. *Journal of Pain and Symptom Management, 36*(6), 559–571. http://doi.org/10.1016/j.jpainsymman.2007.12.018.

Chochinov, H. M., Hassard, T., McClement, S. E., Hack, T., Kristjanson, L. J., Harlos, M., . . . Murray, A. (2009). The landscape of distress in the terminally ill. *Journal of Pain and Symptom Management, 38*(5), 641–649. http://doi.org/10.1016/j.jpainsymman.2009.04.021.

Chochinov, H. M., Kristjanson, L. J., Breitbart, W., McClement, S. E., Hack, T. F., Hassard, T., & Harlos, M. (2011). Effect of dignity therapy on distress and end-of-life experience in terminally ill patients: A randomised controlled trial. *The Lancet Oncology, 12*(8), 753–762. http://doi.org/10.1016/S1470-2045(11)70153-X.

Chochinov, H. M., Kristjanson, L. J., Hack, T. F., Hassard, T., McClement, S. E., & Harlos, M. (2006). Dignity in the terminally ill: Revisited. *Journal of Palliative Medicine, 9*(3), 666–672. http://doi.org/10.1089/jpm.2006.9.666.

Chochinov, H. M., Kristjanson, L. J., Hack, T. F., Hassard, T., McClement, S. E., & Harlos, M. (2007). Burden to others and the terminally ill. *Journal of Pain and*

Symptom Management, 34(5), 463–471. http://doi.org/10.1016/j.jpainsymman.2006.12.012.

Chochinov, H. M., McClement, S. E., Hack, T., Thompson, G., Dufault, B., & Harlos, M. (2014). Eliciting personhood within clinical practice: Effects on patients, families, and health care providers. *Journal of Pain and Symptom Management*, published online, 1–7e2. http://doi.org/10.1016/j.jpainsymman.2014.11.291.

Classen, C., Butler, L. D., Koopman, C, Miller, E., DiMiceli, S., Giese-Davis, J., . . . Spiegel, D. (2001). Supportive-expressive group therapy and distress in patients with metastatic breast cancer: A randomized clinical intervention trial. *Archives of General Psychiatry, 58*(5), 494–501.

Fitchett, G., Emanuel, L., Handzo, G., Boyken, L., & Wilkie, D. J. (2015). Care of the human spirit and the role of dignity therapy: A systematic review of dignity therapy research. *BMC Palliative Care, 14*(8), 1–12. http://doi.org/10.1186/s12904-015-0007-1.

Frankl, V. E. (1966). Self-transcendence as a human phenomenon. *Journal of Humanistic Psychology, 6*, 97–106.

Frankl, V. E. (1984). *Man's search for meaning* (third edition). New York: Pocket Books.

Greer, J. A., Park, E. R., Prigerson, H. G., & Safren, S. A. (2010). Tailoring cognitive-behavioral therapy to treat anxiety comorbid with advanced cancer. *Journal of Cognitive Psychotherapy, 24*(4), 294–313. http://doi.org/10.1891/0889-8391.24.4.294.Tailoring.

Greer, J. A., Traeger, L., Bemis, H., Solis, J., Hendriksen, E. S., Park, E. R., . . . Safren, S. (2012). A pilot randomized controlled trial of brief cognitive-behavioral therapy for anxiety in patients with terminal cancer. *The Oncologist, 17*, 1337–1345.

Greenstein, M., & Breitbart, W. (2000). Cancer and the experience of meaning: A group psychotherapy program for people with cancer. *American Journal of Psychotherapy, 54*, 486–500.

Hack, T. F., McClement, S. E., Chochinov, H. M., Cann, B. J., Hassard, T. H., Kristjanson, L. J., & Harlos, M. (2010). Learning from dying patients during their final days: Life reflections gleaned from dignity therapy. *Palliative Medicine, 24*(7), 715–723. http://doi.org/10.1177/0269216310373164.

Ho, A. H. Y., Leung, P. P. Y., Tse, D. M. W., Pang, S. M. C., Chochinov, H. M., Neimeyer, R. A., & Chan, C. L. W. (2013). Dignity amidst liminality: Healing within suffering among Chinese terminal cancer patients. *Death Studies, 37*(10), 953–970. http://doi.org/10.1080/07481187.2012.703078.

Holland, J., Poppito, S., Nelson, C., Weiss, T., Greenstein, M., Martin, A., . . . Roth, A. (2009). Reappraisal in the eighth life cycle stage: A theoretical psychoeducational intervention in elderly patients with cancer. *Palliative & Supportive Care, 7*(3), 271–279. http://doi.org/10.1017/S1478951509990198.

Kearney, M., & Mount, B. (2000). Spiritual care of the dying patient. In E. Chochinov, M. Harvey, & W. Breitbart (Eds.), *Handbook of psychiatry in palliative medicine* (pp. 357–373). Cary, NC: Oxford University Press.

Kissane, D. W., Block, S., Smith, G. C., Miach, P., Clarke, D. M., Ikin, J., . . . McKenzie, D. (2003). Cognitive-existential group psychotherapy for women with primary breast cancer: A randomised controlled trial. *Psycho-Oncology, 12*(6), 532–546. http://doi.org/10.1002/pon.683.

Kissane, D. W., Grabsch, B., Clarke, D. M., Christie, G., Clifton, D., Gold, S., . . . Smith, G. C. (2004). Supportive-expressive group therapy: The transformation of existential ambivalence into creative living while enhancing adherence to anti-cancer therapies. *Psycho-Oncology, 13*(11), 755–768. http://doi.org/10.1002/pon.798.

Kissane, D. W., Grabsch, B., Clarke, D. M., Smith, G. C., Love, A. W., Bloch, S., . . . Li, Y. (2007). Supportive-expressive group therapy for women with metastatic breast cancer: Survival and psychosocial outcome from a randomized controlled trial. *Psycho-Oncology, 16*, 277–286. http://doi.org/10.1002/pon.

Lo, C., Hales, S., Jung, J., Chiu, A., Panday, T., Rydall, A., . . . Rodin, G. (2014). Managing Cancer And Living Meaningfully (CALM): Phase 2 trial of a brief individual psychotherapy for patients with advanced cancer. *Palliative Medicine, 28*(3), 234–242. http://doi.org/10.1177/0269216313507757.

McClement, S. E, Chochinov, H. M., Hack, T., Hassard, T., Kristjanson, L. J., & Harlos, M. (2007). Dignity therapy: Family member perspectives. *Journal of Palliative Medicine, 10*(5), 1076–1082. http://doi.org/10.1089/jpm.2007.0002.

McClement, S. E., Chochinov, H. M., Hack, T. F., Kristjanson, L. J., & Harlos, M. (2004). Dignity conserving care: Application of research findings to practice. *International Journal of Palliative Nursing, 10*(4), 173–179.

Mclean, L. M., Walton, T., Rodin, G., Esplen, M. J., & Jones, J. M. (2013). A couple-based intervention for patients and caregivers facing end-stage cancer: Outcomes of a randomized controlled trial. *Psycho-Oncology, 22*(1), 28–38.

Montross, L., Winters, K. D., & Irwin, S. A. (2011). Dignity therapy implementation in a community-based hospice setting. *Journal of Palliative Medicine, 14*(6), 729–734. http://doi.org/10.1089/jpm.2010.0449.

Nissim, R., Freeman, E., Lo, C., Zimmermann, C., Gagliese, L., Rydall, A., . . . Rodin, G. (2012). Managing cancer and living meaningfully (CALM): A qualitative study of a brief individual psychotherapy for individuals with advanced cancer. *Palliative Medicine, 26*(5), 713–721. http://doi.org/10.1177/0269216311425096.

Proulx, K. (2004). Dying with dignity: The good patient versus the good death. *American Journal of Hospice & Palliative Medicine, 21*(2), 116–120. http://doi.org/10.1177/104990910402100209.

Southwick, S. M., Gilmartin, R., McDonough, P., & Morrissey, P. (2006). Logotherapy as an adjunctive treatment for chronic combat-related PTSD: A meaning-based intervention. *American Journal of Psychotherapy, 60*(2), 161–174. Retrieved from www.ncbi.nlm.nih.gov/pubmed/16892952.

Steinhauser, K. E., Alexander, S. C., Byock, I. R., George, L. K., & Tulsky, J. A. (2009). Seriously ill patients' discussions of preparation and life completion: An intervention to assist with transition at the end of life. *Palliative & Supportive Care, 7*(4), 393–404. http://doi.org/10.1017/S147895150999040X.

Van Gennip, I. E., Pasman, H.R.W., Kaspers, P. J., Oosterveld-Vlug, M. G., Willems, D. L., Deeg, D.J.H., & Onwuteaka-Philipsen, B. D. (2013). Death with dignity from the perspective of the surviving family: A survey study among family caregivers of deceased older adults. *Palliative Medicine, 27*(7), 616–624. http://doi.org/10.1177/0269216313483185.

Whitford, H. S., & Olver, I. N. (2012). The multidimensionality of spiritual wellbeing: Peace, meaning, and faith and their association with quality of life and coping in oncology. *Psycho-Oncology, 21*, 602–610.

Part III

Characterizing the Concept of the Good Death

8 What Promise Exists for a Good Death?

> What value is there in the last phase of life? Can there be any mean-
> ing and value in the process of dying? Can there be value in grieving?
> Can there be value in caring for people as they die?
>
> (Byock 2002, p. 285)

Is there such a thing as a good death? If so, what are the elements of a good
death, in contrast to a death filled with torment and desolation? In spite of
much attention paid to the concept since the middle of the 20th century,
a good death remained more of a hope than a standard of medical care
by the time Emanuel and Emanuel's (1998) classic study of the question,
The Promise of a Good Death, examined various parameters of the concept in depth. In a death-denying culture, fueled by a search for youth, by
lengthening life-spans, by lower childhood mortality, smaller families, and
the increase in use of medical technology, a positive ideal of a good death
was elusive. Chapter 8 briefly examines the issues of the Right to Die debate,
which some individuals consider to be a good death, and then explores the
emerging attributes of the good death construct as expressed by patients,
families, caregivers, doctors, researchers, and scholars.

8.1 THE RIGHT TO DIE: SUICIDE, EUTHANASIA, PHYSICIAN-ASSISTED SUICIDE (PAS), AND THE GOOD DEATH

> Although palliative care is publicly against active voluntary eutha-
> nasia, the two actually have one important feature in common.
> Both find support in individualistic societies that promote personal
> autonomy—the right of individuals to make their own choices about
> how they should live and die. For advocates of both palliative care
> and euthanasia, the good death is one in which I make my own
> choices about my last days and months.
>
> (Walter, 2003, p. 219)

The issue of euthanasia has been debated vigorously and publicly in the Netherlands since the early 1970s. The "right to die" debate in the United States in the early 2000s impacted on the growing legions of the terminal elderly who no longer wanted to bear the physical and psychosocial pain of the end of life. The "right to die" lobby campaigned for painless, easy death that represented the inalienable human right to self-determination and culminated in the "Natural Death" legislation enacted in the state of Oregon in the United States and the legalization of voluntary euthanasia in the Netherlands. The rise in suicide and requests for physician-assisted suicide (PAS) contributed to turning the full attention of the U.S. government to ways of improving end-of-life care, using the prior knowledge gained from research studies. The physical and psychosocial needs of terminally ill patients became clear but means of addressing them in order to improve the quality of end-of-life care were just beginning to emerge. Healthcare professionals sought to determine how to "take a more proactive, rather than reactive, approach to end-of-life care that prevents suffering or addresses it before it spins out of control" (Schroepfer, 2007, pp. 136–7). The events common to the dying process—pain, loss of autonomy, loss of social support, depression, loss of independence, poor quality of life, loss of meaning in life, loss of interest or pleasure in activities, hopelessness, drowsiness, weakness, loss of control, and high caregiving needs—had to be identified and implemented in order to provide comfort for the terminal elderly that made hastening the ends of their lives less attractive (Schroepfer, 2007). However, refractory symptoms may arise that complicate or obviate the relief of pain, forcing physicians to a decision to use terminal sedation, wherein dying individuals with such unendurable pain are kept in a deep state of sleep. In this situation, deaths that are known to be imminent and unavoidable may be hastened slightly as a foreseen but unintentional by-product of the drugs administered (Seymour et al., 2002, p. 290). Whether or not this practice is legal—"killing" or "letting die"—is a topic of considerable debate in palliative care circles.

The terms "euthanasia" and "physician-assisted suicide" are two different concepts: the term euthanasia, from the Greek words *eu thanatos* meaning "good death", means "voluntary active euthanasia"; that is, the physician intentionally ends the patient's life at the patient's request and with the patient's full informed consent. "Physician-assisted suicide" (PAS) refers to the physician's act of providing medication, a prescription, information, or other interventions to a patient with the understanding that the patient intends to use them to commit suicide (Ward & Tate, 1994). PAS is legal in the Netherlands, Belgium, and Switzerland. In the United States, Oregon legalized PAS in 1997, the practice was legalized in Washington State in March of 2009, and in Vermont in May 2013. Both euthanasia and PAS are practiced globally, albeit at a very low rate. The majority of requests for each of these methods have come from those who have cancer (Emanuel & Fairclough, 1996).

In most reports, uncontrolled pain is not a major determinant of interest in or use of euthanasia or PAS (Meier et al., 1998; Emanuel & Fairclough, 1996; Emanuel et al., 1998; Wilson et al., 2000). In a report of the Death with Dignity program at the Fred Hutchinson/University of Washington Cancer Consortium in Washington state, the most common reasons for pursuing PAS were loss of autonomy (97 percent), inability to engage in enjoyable activities (89 percent), and loss of dignity (75 percent); only 22 percent had concerns about inadequate pain control (Loggers et al., 2013). Breitbart et al. (1996) studied the interest in PAS amongst HIV-infected patients and found that the strongest predictors of this interest were psychological distress, being of Caucasian race, infrequent or no attendance at religious services, and perceived low levels of psychosocial support (p. 238). These findings support the reports of psychiatric and social factors rather than physical ones as causes of requests for PAS.

Many rationales exist for each side of the debate regarding the right to die or the lack thereof, but extensive review of each side is beyond the scope of this book. Suffice it to say that each side of the argument might well insist that the evidence on their particular view would provide the scenario for a good death. Many rationales support the legalization of the right to die, however that may be achieved. Given the circumstances of increasing pain and disability and burden to others, the decision to end one's life may seem rational (Breitbart & Rosenfeld, 1999). Those patients who have relied upon their physicians during the course of their illness, may feel that PAS is the natural end point to the relationship. However, a main concern of physicians dealing with such a request was found to be failing to detect a treatable depression or some other kind of mood disorder (Deschepper et al., 2014, p. 617). Also, pain-relieving medication is all too available to those suffering from a terminal illness. Opponents of the legalization of the many forms of the right to die, logically begin with the Hippocratic Oath taken by each person who becomes a physician. Physicians are sworn to heal and to extend life, however most surveys find that the majority of American physicians oppose euthanasia and PAS (Emanuel & Fairclough, 1996; Meier et al., 1998).

Depressive symptoms, hopelessness, and other psychological factors are consistently associated with interest in PAS and euthanasia. Depression, hopelessness, and helplessness are the dominant presenting psychological symptoms of terminally ill individuals who seek to hasten death, as well as unrelieved pain and symptom control, and lack of social support. The oncologic psychiatrists have found that controlling depression with appropriate targeting of psychopharmaceuticals can improve many of the reasons for hastening death (Breitbart & Rosenfeld, 1999; Chochinov et al., 1998; Wilson et al., 2000).

A 2013 systematic international literature review (Hendry et al.) aimed to shed light on the perspectives of ordinary people about assisted dying, when they are ill or disabled. A key construct is unbearable suffering and four themes were revealed relating to the reasons for and against pursuing assisted dying or allowing its use: concerns about poor quality of life including unbearable suffering, dependency, burden and loss of self, physical pain and suffering, and fear of future suffering; concerns about abuse if assisted dying were legalized—the need for safeguards, the influence of financial pressure, vulnerable groups and discrimination, and the role of others in decision making; the importance of individual stance related to assisted dying, such as moral or religious views, personal experience of death or suffering, being for or against the availability or legalization of assisted dying; and the desire for a good quality of death by virtue of autonomy and control and the right time to die. As previously noted in prior empirical studies, "unbearable suffering relating to psycho-emotional factors such as hopelessness, feeling a burden, loss of interest or pleasure and loneliness were at least as significant as pain and other physical symptoms in motivating people to consider assisted dying" (Hendry et al., 2013, p. 23) stood out as major concerns. Regardless of health status, the right to choose and the desire for autonomy with regard to the manner of death was a good death theme (Wilson et al., 2000) expressed in most of the reviewed studies.

In a 2006 investigation regarding the experience of dying, patients close to death were interviewed regarding the desire to shorten their lives (Terry et al.). Each patient claimed to have had entertained thoughts about doing so, ranging from fleeting thoughts that life was not worth living, or had gone on long enough, through the expressed wish that they were dead or an isolating preoccupation with death to communicating a plan or a well-reasoned course of action for suicide (p. 383). When asked why they did not kill themselves, the reason for not acting on the desire to hasten death that was most frequently stated was not the sense that doing so was wrong but the uncertainty about their ability to end their life without increased suffering or without implicating others in illegalities (p. 384). Secondly, another group of reasons for not committing suicide concerned the reactions to their act of those left behind would. These patients were not concerned about the justifiability of suicide in their own minds. Their decisive concerns were about how the people they left behind would interpret their actions.

David Lester (2006) raised the issue of suicide being considered a good death by dividing the question into two parts: whether suicide can be considered an appropriate death or a rational death. Lester discussed Weisman's proposition that an appropriate death must fulfill four criteria, which will be discussed in greater detail below. Lester claimed that in fulfilling each of these criteria for an appropriate death, "a suicidal death could be deemed appropriate" (p. 512).

Likewise, Lester proposed that a death from natural causes without medical intrusion may be viewed as appropriate; that an individual who dies in a manner that is consistent with his or her lifestyle may be said to have died an appropriate death; that suicide could be considered an appropriate death when it was a timely death (2006, pp. 514–16). Lester then considered whether a rational death could be a good death, wherein "rationality refers to the reasonableness of the premises or assumptions that are used in arguing for or justifying a decision" (p. 517). Lester then considered various criteria considered reasonable for determining the rationality of a suicide and the ability therefore of considering suicide rational and therefore a good death.

Self-destructive desires are perhaps most understandable when expressed by elderly people. This segment of population may be motivated by feelings of meaninglessness, loneliness, worthlessness, and helplessness; the loss of roles and of significant others; and by depression that dampen the desire to live. These issues in end-of-life care are increasingly being brought to the public's attention. People are becoming aware of the institutionalization of elderly individuals that spells out for them the loss of control leading to loss of dignity.

In an analysis of Belgian newspaper articles on medical end-of-life decision making, Van Brussel and Carpentier (2012, in Semino et al., 2014, p. 669) discuss more specifically the discursive construction of a good death in the north Belgian 2008 press coverage of three euthanasia cases. The authors suggest that the notion of a good death has been politicized, particularly in the discourses associated with palliative care on the one hand and the right to die on the other. The palliative care movement associates a good death with control, autonomy, and dignity, in contrast to the right-to-die movement that associates it with awareness and heroism, and suggest that this politicization of death, whether good or bad, can affect the range of acceptable choices that patients and families are presented with.

8.2 ANALYSES OF THE GOOD DEATH FROM STAKEHOLDERS' PERSPECTIVES

> What does it mean for patients to say they want to die with dignity, or quietly, or suddenly? What is the meaning of the desire for death? Does suffering have any meaning? How do these notions vary across cultures, time, and space?
>
> (Clark, 2003, p. 174)

Hundreds of journal articles as well as dozens of books having to do with good death concepts were identified and studied while researching this book. The articles and books were written by physicians, nurses, and other providers, from both large and small institutions and research laboratories, by sociologists, anthropologists, historians, ethnographers, thanatologists, ethicists, psychiatrists, psychologists, and philosophers from their own research or experiential perspectives or from those of patients, families, caregivers, theologists. Each of those professionals researched, interviewed, tested, analyzed, and wrote about the ideology, ideals, ideas, notions, connotations, factors, domains, and theories of death concepts applicable to the good death. This attempt to define and characterize the term good death was accompanied as well by the otherwise adjectively modified words pertaining to death that were presented at the very beginning of this book. The upshot? All findings boil down to roughly the same definitions, ideas, concepts, notions, or qualifications of the good death, representing a "cultural script that is dominant in the international literature of palliative care" (Goldsteen et al., 2006, p. 379). Much of this material is summarized and presented in this chapter.

Walter (2003) compared the difference between the good deaths as narrated by Ariès and those of today's societies: in the 19th century in rural France, the priest was first called to the bedside, but today the doctor is, illustrating that religion was then the influence, as opposed to that of medicine today. In the earlier time, each person knew their role in the proceedings of death; today palliative care encourages patients to formulate their own role. In the 19th century the patient was expected to die in a matter of days, while today, in our ultra-globalized, ultra-individualized world, we take years to die, often in hospital surrounded by technology and strangers instead of at home surrounded by family/friends. Today the community does not dictate the choice of religion, the individual does, while seeking answers and support from other patients on the internet. Within a multicultural society, norms for a good death vary widely (Walter, 2003, p. 218). In the 19th century, medical skills were called upon as a matter secondary to the religious aim of bringing the dying person into a right relationship with God (Walters, 2004).

The second half of the 20th century saw advances in biomedical technology focused on the concept of the good death as a fight against disease. The modern hospice movement emerged and redefined a good death as one that included acceptance and closure as a determinant of quality in end-of-life care (Costello, 2006). In Costello's (2006) study using focus groups with physicians, the healthcare providers emphasized biomedical issues, reinforcing the fact that death for this segment is viewed mostly through the lens of biomedical explanation wherein death is primarily defined as a physiologic event. However, as time has passed, a strictly biomedical perspective has proven incomplete, because the concept of death today operates additionally from the psychosocial perspective that considers death as a part of life rather than a failure of technology (Steinhauser, Christakis, et al., 2000; Steinhauser, Clipp, et al., 2000).

The Issue of End-of-Life Preferences and Decision Making on Good Death

The medical imperative that dying people should be free of pain and other intolerable symptoms has been standard in Western societies, particularly with the advent of palliative care. However, practical problems emerged in Western countries from palliative care's ability to control pain: the need to balance this clinical expertise with the ethical issues of autonomy, self-determination, and awareness. Thus, having a voice in the decision-making process and in the choice of medical treatments has frequently been recognized as important to achieving a good death.

The ability to make decisions about one's own dying and death is commonly considered a necessary component of a good death (Balducci, 2012, iii59). The wishes of the patients, if they are able to voice them, as well as those of the families or surrogates, if they are not, must be considered. Obtaining care consistent with patient's wishes is related to the degree to which patients communicate with their physicians. A "therapeutic alliance" between doctor and patient is advantageous in achieving the desired outcome (Mack et al., 2010, p. 1204).

The practice of modern palliative care has sought to promote the autonomy of patients and caregivers and to facilitate the collaboration between patient/caregivers and their clinicians. Participants in a British study (Seymour et al., 2002) concerning older peoples' assessments of the risks and benefits of end-of-life care "understood an *idealised* death to be that in which morphine administration and terminal sedation serve to provide dying people with an easy, comfortable and quiet death" (p. 287). The risks and benefits were seen to depend on moral and social concerns. Thus, Seymour et al. found that patients and caregivers were accorded a position of ultimate authority, with clinicians functioning as co-experts in order to negotiate the best possible quality of life for dying people and to achieve a good death.

For Dutch citizens, accepting euthanasia, terminal sedation, and the use of high dosages of morphine were associated with the wish to have a *dignified death* and with concerns about burdening loved ones with terminal care. A study investigating the preferences of the Dutch general public (Rietjens et al., 2006) identified dying a pain-free and dignified death, having the possibility to say goodbye to loved ones, and being able to personally decide about end-of-life treatments as the main priorities. To the Dutch, acceptance of euthanasia was also associated with the wish to achieve some sense of control of medical end-of-life treatments (Rietjens et al., 2006).

Terry et al.'s (2006) study concerned another aspect of end-of-life preferences: often the preferences of the dying patient differed from those of families or carers. The patients sought privacy and autonomy, timely, relevant information, and the desire to shorten their life. The carer group was also concerned with lacking information about the patient's illness, of recognition of their role as carer, of their difficulty interpreting the emotional and physical changes associated with dying, and of the difficulty obtaining practical help (Terry et al., 2006, p. 340). Many of these preferences put the wishes of the two groups in direct opposition to each other in terms of autonomy, privacy, and decision making. The study pointed out the philosophy of hospice that considered the family as the unit of care and thereby created tension about information-sharing: some patients saw in this a violation of their privacy should they not want to share personal information with their family; patients wanted the autonomy to make their own treatment decisions and not to be forced into sharing their very personal thoughts about their imminent death. Carers, however, felt they needed information in order to fulfill their caring role. The motivation for increased information often concerned the process of dying. Patients were concerned that they "might in their final moments behave in a way that was out of character or bizarre and they were anxious to be told if this was likely" (p. 342), a part of their desire to maintain their self-image and to spare the family distress. Both groups were interested in knowing about events that might signify impending death, but the carer group also wanted to understand the moods and anger of the patient in order to be of most help.

Perspectives and Preferences from the Providers' Points of View

The good death concept was central to hospice philosophy and emerged as a reaction to the medicalization and bureaucratization of death and dying. The good death has become central to sustaining hospice care against increasing threats and challenges (Hart et al., 1998, p. 70). McNamara et al.'s (1995) studies concluded that nurses and other health professionals were working hard to uphold the principles of the good death while at the same time acknowledging that such an ideal was difficult to attain.

These studies examined how hospice nurses in Australia developed shared strategies and logic to cope with the extraordinary stress imposed on them by their role as professional caregivers to the terminally ill. The hospice model, delivering patient-centered holistic care, was seen to "challenge the mainstream medical model by offering an alternative, better way to die" (McNamara et al., 1995, p. 223). The nurse's ability to cope is based on developing a shared strategy supplying meaning and direction that is built upon the hospice philosophy. The good death model, derived from sociological, anthropological, and psychological perspectives, is therefore defined as good if the patient demonstrates awareness, acceptance, and preparation for death. If the patient is to have a good death, nurses feel that they should: "ideally be involved; provide effective symptom control so that the patient may complete their living and die pain free; and work toward providing an environment where the patient may die peacefully and with dignity" (McNamara et al., 1995, p. 224).

As demonstrated in two studies (Low & Payne, 1996; Payne et al., 1996), the caring behavior of palliative care nurses was shown to be determined by their perceptions of good/bad deaths: they viewed the circumstances of good death as the control of the physical symptoms of the patient's illness and the ability of being open with the patient about the nature of his or her prognosis (Costello, 2006). Conversely, a bad death was one in which the patient's physical discomforts went uncontrolled and the diagnosis of the impending death was not accepted. The palliative care nurses and social workers believed that a good death involved patients being at peace with themselves (Masson, 2002), living life to the full and dying in a place of their choice with people close to them at the time of death. Their aim was to ensure death without discomfort, physically or psychologically, views that seem to echo Sudnow's ideas of the patient's and family's "negotiation and acceptance of end of life circumstances" (in Low & Payne, 1996, p. 238). In a separate study, Payne, Langley-Evans, and Hillier (1996) showed that patients' views of a good death differed from those of nurses: patients specified as preferable "dying in one's sleep, dying quietly, with dignity, being pain free and dying suddenly" (p. 307).

The findings of a study of a sample of registered nurses working in an acute medical wards seems similar to McNamara et al. (1995) in defining how the nurses developed a common, shared strategy when working with dying patients. The nurses concluded that a death could be considered an ideal death if the patient was peaceful, dignified, and comfortable; the death had to be an expected death with someone in the room at the point of death. The nurses' perceptions of the good death were often differentiated from each other, suggesting that "shared and personal values combined to shaped individual nurses understanding of a good death" (Hopkinson & Hallett, 2002, p. 538).

Griggs (2010) identified many challenges associated with the provision of end-of-life care that contributed to a good death in this setting, the major difficulty being that "75% of the week falls outside of normal working hours" (p. 146), complicating access to drugs for off-hour nurses. A purposive sample of community nurses participated in qualitative research to identify the necessary components of a good death in the community. The list of themes (see Table 3 in Griggs, 2010, p. 142) identified as important to community nurses began with symptom control motivated by patient comfort and dignity; patient choice due to respect for patient wishes; the need for honesty, openness, awareness; spirituality contributing to peace; interprofessional relationships entailed the efficiency and ability of health professionals to work together to ensure a good death; the need for formal handover was a need for communication; preparation and organization represented by prescribing practices, availability of resources, and anticipatory planning; and seamless care to cover out of hours care.

In two other care environments, studies of the components of a good death revealed results that were relatively similar to those of Payne et al. (1996) and Steinhauser, Christakis, et al. (2000). Hodde et al. (2004) (as cited in Coombs & Long, 2008, p. 210) reported that a "quality death for critical care nurses working in ICUs is associated with establishment of a diagnosis, the nurse/family being present at the time of death, withdrawal of life support and no resuscitation measures instituted 8 hours prior to death" (as cited in Coombs & Long, 2008, p. 210). Nurses working in the long-term care of nursing homes (Gibson et al., 2008) surveyed the opinions of healthcare providers about the relative importance of 20 attributes of a good death: twelve survey items were identified by the majority of respondents as essential or important to a good death, including "symptom control items and items relating to the psychosocial and spiritual aspects of death" (Gibson et al., 2008, p. 378).

The care environment specifically of in-hospice experiences was explored in a 2010 Australian sociological study focusing on what the patients there experienced as a good death. The study revealed a diverse set of preferences, including personal and interpersonal tensions around what was considered a good death, struggle talk, the desire for the end that was not messy for relatives, and achievement of peace and calmness in the final moments (Broom & Cavenagh, 2010, p. 871). The authors argued that death in a hospice is shaped by the presence of normative understandings of the good death but also complex personal and biographical factors (p. 874).

Semino et al. (2014) explored the formal and functional characteristics of narratives of good and bad deaths as told by 13 British hospice managers to illustrate what they saw as a good or a bad death. The narratives revealed the role of hospices and their professional staff in facilitating good death. The interviewees described a good death primarily in terms of peacefulness, symptom control, frank conversations, acceptance, and openness to physical and emotional support. Conversely, they had described a bad death primarily in terms of "conflict within families, lack of acceptance, rejection of physical and emotional support, and physical and emotional distress" (p. 681).

Physicians usually do not refer to their patient's clinical situation by using the terms "good death" or "bad death". Instead, they use narrative to characterize the quality of both the patients and their own experience, showing that the process of dying is not easy, not a simple matter of good or bad death. Three major themes of the physicians' narratives emerged that framed their positive and negative experiences: Time and Process indicating whether the death was expected or unexpected, peaceful, chaotic, or prolonged; Medical Care and Treatment Decisions regarding whether end-of-life care was rational and appropriate, facilitating a peaceful or gentle death, or futile and overly aggressive, fraught with irrational decisions or adverse events; and Communication and Negotiation concerning whether communication with patients, family, and medical teams was effective, leading to satisfying management of end-of-life care, or characterized by misunderstandings and conflict (DelVecchio Good et al., 2004, p. 939). Much thought and discussion clearly went into the decisions facing these doctors.

Patients' Perspectives

Technology and biomedicine extended life expectancy and improved how diseases were treated. For many individuals death is considered a function of old age, a failure of medicine to hinder the inevitable, or as a process to be prevented or prolonged. Individuals are often loathe to discuss their views of death, including their own, and when necessary to do so, employ euphemisms such as pass away, sleep, and rest to soften the effect of their words. The term "good death" evolved from the hospice movement and helped to minimize the fear associated with perceptions of death (Hughes et al., 2008, p. 39). Some researchers point out that the needs of patients that indicate their preferences for end-of-life care are not as highly represented as other stakeholders. The following research from the various perspectives of patients attempts to clarify perceptions of a good death.

Kellehear studied advanced cancer patients in their last year of life and identified the key features of a good death as involving much social interaction and comprising: (1) the social life of the dying person; (2) the creation of open awareness; (3) the social adjustment to and personal preparation for death; (4) the public preparations such as arrangements relating to work; and (5) the final farewells (Kellehear, 1990, in Payne et al., 1996, p. 308). Kellehear concluded that the good death is good in two senses: "at the individual level in a psychological sense as it gives the dying person opportunities for order and control, and . . . at the social level as it provides a series of rites for appropriate disengagement" (cited in Hart et al., 1998, p. 71).

Vig et al.'s (2002) study of non-terminally ill older adults' perceptions of good and bad death was distinguished by the heterogeneity of responses. These ill patients revealed that the preferred means of death would be in one's sleep and, conversely, that prolonged dying produced a bad death. Other responses indicated that a good death would be quick, painless, without suffering, peaceful, at peace with God, without having knowledge of their impending death; a bad death was seen as painful, prolonged, dependent (on machines), causing suffering, burdening others, and shortness of breath. In this sample of non-terminally ill adults some homogeneity of study results exists but the majority of them held heterogeneous views despite similar baseline characteristics.

A qualitative study of people 80 years or older dwelling in the community that explored their perceptions on death, dying, and end of life care reflected that a good death for this population would be death that involves the minimum amount of physical or mental dependency/disability, minimum amount of being a burden to others, and one that involved staying in their own home (Lloyd-Williams et al., 2007, p. 64).

The objective of a study from the perspective of patients with advanced AIDS was to identify and describe the domains defining what they viewed as a good versus bad death (Pierson et al., 2002). The patients were asked to describe a good and bad death. Analyses of the responses revealed 12 domains describing their concerns: symptoms—the absence of pain indicated good death, while presence of pain indicated bad death; quality of life—indicated the need to be in a comfortable state, without suffering and not having prolonged dying via life support; people present—most, but not all, participants felt that having loved ones present was an important concern; dying process—respondents were concerned about various aspects of the process of dying, such as their death being a drawn out process, the hope for death to happen while sleeping, or for dying to be "like drifting off to sleep" (p. 591); issues of location of death—very important to having a good death, eliciting various opinions of death in hospital, in a hospice, or at home for a good death, while the opposite opinions of those options were also mentioned by many; a sense of resolution—having a good death entailed dying without unresolved issues or unanswered questions, having said goodbyes, having time to prepare for death and, for many, "feeling at peace both with self and others" (p. 592); patient control of treatment—the need for a sense of control in decision-making; issues of spirituality—some of the respondents indicated the necessity of spiritual matter to a good death; death scene—in order to shape a good death, quiet and no crying were important; physician-assisted suicide—some participants voiced the desire for PAS to be an option; aspects of medical care—patients felt the importance to a good death of having access to the medical care they needed, having a good relationship with their physician, being treated as an individual or a whole person by their physician and caregivers, and feeling they were receiving quality medical care; and acceptance of death—that they could not have a good death unless they had accepted the death. A number of these domains had previously been included in the results of end-of-life studies and several extended beyond the scope of medicine. However, being familiar with these concerns would assist physicians to know their patients' preferences.

A 2003 study (Tong et al.) of the perceptions of a good death among minority and non-minority community dwellers confirmed the attributes of a good death as recognized by most researchers. The minority group was composed predominantly of people of color or of less common religious affiliations such as Buddhists or Muslims; the non-minority group consisted of people of Judeo-Christian or European background. Each of the groups presented a collection of similar views of a good death; however, three areas of difference between the two groups were also recognized: domains of spiritual concerns, of cultural concerns, and of individuation. Both groups spoke of the importance to them of spiritual concerns, but the non-minority group expressed that their needs for appropriate spiritual care and religious practices were lacking; the minority group believed that inequity in access to spiritual care existed. Minority groups felt that healthcare providers did not facilitate important cultural traditions for them in end-of-life care. Both groups discussed the importance of individuation but their fears about lacking individuation differed in their sources: non-minority participants feared losing desired independence and personal autonomy and that individuation would be compromised by persistent stereotyping based on their race or ethnicity. The findings may help to encourage more culturally sensitive and humane end-of-life care for both minority and non-minority individuals, as well as smoothing the path towards dying well for them.

A study addressing the deaths of patients and the resultant psychological distress suffered by the spouses (Carr, 2003), investigated the premise that a good death is less distressing for the patient than for the families, as well as questioning the knowledge base of how frequent the good death occurs and the factors that may predict who will experience it. Carr suggested that, while the typical markers indicating a good death is upheld as an ideal, death quality may instead be linked to death cause or to its suddenness. Likewise, Carr sought a correlation between the quality of a spouse's death and the psychological distress of the survivor, six months post-death. Analyses revealed that the cause, suddenness, and timing of the death best predict the objective characteristics of the death. Predictors of the surviving spouse's psychological distress are indicated by the dying patient's medical care and the interactions between decedent and survivors. Religious beliefs affect both how the survivors interpret their spouses' final days and their psychological health following the loss. Carr proposed that the analyses indicate that there may be two paths to the good death: "sudden deaths are less painful for the decedent but hinder the spouses ability to discuss and understand the process of death" (p. 225). Three aspects of the death considered critical—having led a full life, accepting one's impending death, and not being burdensome to family members—prove to be unrelated to the level of the spouse's psychological distress. The explanation of these conclusions may be that the psychological stress created by caregiving may be balanced by rewards such as increased closeness with an ill spouse and a heightened sense of purpose (p. 226). Religious beliefs appear to protect the bereaved from high levels of anger and to influence the survivors' appraisals of the dying process. In contrast, although persons who die of terminal illnesses have the time to discuss their death with family members and to resolve unfinished psychological and practical business, they also are more likely to "experience pain and discomfort" (p. 216). The effects of cognitive impairment, dementia or delirium also contribute to the inability of the dying to communicate such preferences to the survivors, and so decrease the possibility of a good death. The conclusion that the "idealized good death may be impossible to achieve" (p. 217) appears to be reasonable in light of the analyses, but appear to provide an interesting view about the losses suffered by the bereaved.

Terms Used to Define a Good Death

> Death is feared, all thoughts of it are avoided and the dying themselves are often left in loneliness. Both in their homes and in hospital, they are emotionally isolated even when surrounded by their families or involved in much therapeutic activity. . . . The last stages of life should not be seen as defeat, but rather as life's fulfillment.
>
> (Saunders, 1965, p. 70)

The good death concept is characterized by its *attributes*. Most of the common attributes of a good death have been defined by healthcare providers and families/caregivers, fewer by patients themselves. The attributes named in the following text will be mostly from the patients' points of view and will vary depending on the subjective views of each of these stakeholder groups.

Steinhauser et al.'s early clinical research on the good death concept set the standards for defining the concept. In the classic study conducted in 2000 by Steinhauser, Clipp, et al., which was significant for including information from dying patients, as well as from healthcare providers and caregivers, most participants cited as their number one priority in defining a good death the wish not to die in pain or to suffer breakthrough of pain or unrelieved dyspnea (air hunger). The participants identified six major components of a good death that are process-oriented attributes of a good death, each possessing biomedical, psychological, social, and spiritual components (Steinhauser, Clipp, et al., 2000, p. 827, from Table 3):

1. Pain and symptom management: participants feared dying in pain.
2. Clear decision making: fear of pain could be reduced through communication and clear decision making with physicians.
3. Preparation for death: to know what to expect during their illness; to plan for events that would follow their death; not precluding elements of hope.
4. Completion: includes faith issues, life review, resolving conflicts, spending time with family and friends, saying good-bye.
5. Contributing to others: desire to contribute to others' well-being (gifts, time, knowledge).
6. Affirmation of the whole person: affirming the person as a unique and whole person.

Most patients cited as their number one priority in defining a good death the wish not to die in pain or to suffer breakthrough of pain or unrelieved dyspnea (air hunger). Psychological distress contributes to physical symptoms and experiencing pain undermines coping ability and is a threat to the integrity of self (Block, 2001). Patients understood that such fears could be reduced by clear communication and by participating in their care with shared decision making, a criterion that empowered patients. The need to understand what would happen to them along the trajectory of their illness was important to patients in terms of completing wills, making funeral arrangements, and writing obituaries. Caregivers expressed the need for a sense of what physical and psychosocial changes could be expected. Study participants sought a sense of completion, marked not only by faith issues, but also by life review, resolution of conflicts, and spending time with family and friends in order to say goodbye. Patients valued being viewed as persons rather than as their disease (Steinhauser, Christakis, et al., 2000; Steinhauser, Clipp, et al., 2000). Patients and families characterized a bad death as one lacking the opportunity to plan ahead, to arrange personal affairs, to decrease family burden, or to say goodbye.

In a separate study, Steinhauser et al. (2001) explored the importance to all patients of being prepared for the end of life and knowing that one's family is prepared. Respondents from all groups also showed consensus on the importance of five other components of preparation: "naming someone to make decisions, knowing what to expect about one's physical condition, having financial affairs in order, having treatment preferences in writing, and knowing that one's physician is comfortable talking about death and dying" (p. 730).

The results of Steinhauser's focus groups in the 2000 studies showed both strong agreement and variation among participants. The first four themes amongst the six major ones identified were elements that were common to the philosophy of palliative care; however, a new criterion was found, centering on the need of patients to contribute to others in some way (Steinhauser, Christakis, et al., 2000; Steinhauser, Clipp, et al., 2000). Such a criterion balances the acceptance of help from others at the end of life, minimizes the sense of being a burden, and produces a beneficial feeling of self-*transcendence* (Coward & Reed, 1996). This desire to reciprocate speaks to Erikson's concept of generativity (1982) that is also a factor in Chochinov's Dignity Protocol (Chochinov et al., 2013). The study also highlighted an important difference between the healthcare provider segment and the patient/family group: the need to attend to aspects of care that are not intuitively important to clinicians but are critical to patients and their families, such as physicians being more willing than patients to sacrifice lucidity for pain control, even though patients placed a great deal of importance on being mentally aware. Patients and families tended to view the end of life with broader psychosocial and spiritual meaning. Lastly, patients highly valued attention to spirituality, particularly, the importance of coming to peace with God and praying (Steinhauser, Christakis, et al., 2000, p. 2481).

Beginning in the 1990s, Chochinov's clinical research established the concept of dignity that emerged as a required attribute of good death. The concept of dignity in dying represents the unconditional quality of human worth, but also the "external qualities of physical comfort, autonomy, meaningfulness, usefulness, preparedness, spirituality and interpersonal connection, and dying at home" (Proulx & Jacelon (2004, p. 116). In their literature review, Proulx and Jacelon's views on the good death ideology are consistent with those of McNamara (2004), Walter (2003), and Masson (2002), with the added measure of the need for dignity in death. Christakis (2007, p. 201) presented three aspects of dignified care at the end of life that are closely related to those of good death:

1. bodily concerns (such as cognitive acuity, functional capacity, physical and psychological distress);
2. dignity practices (such as the ability to help others, being hopeful, maintaining a sense of normalcy); and
3. social features (such as not burdening others, being concerned about the aftermath of one's death, and having social support).

However, the concept of human dignity is essentially violated by the default choice of technology when the patient becomes distressed, which results in the prescribing of life-prolonging treatment until death. A corollary of violating a patient's dignity by unwanted prolongation of life is often the individual's desire for hastened death.

In Kehl's (2006) literature review that analyzed the concept of the good death, she cited O'Neill (1983) as having made the first attempt at defining a good death. According to her research, during the 1960s and 1970s, the term "good death" was used as a synonym to imply euthanasia, when lives were ended either actively or passively. Kehl claimed that since O'Neill was primarily discussing the situations that needed to be present for appropriate euthanasia to occur, the definition also appropriately applied to the term good death. O'Neill defined death as good if the "timing of the death is appropriate, the dying process allows the person to retain control, those involved in the dying situation observe basic moral principles, and the death style of the person is logical" (in Kehl, 2006, p. 278).

In Kehl's analysis of the literature review on defining good death between 1966 and 2004, death is most often characterized as being "highly individual, changeable over time, and based on perspective and experience" (p. 281), with some disagreement about whether death was an event or process, such that the quality of dying may change over time during the process (see Proulx, 2004). Kehl (2006, p. 281) identified agreement on the following attributes of a good death:

> . . . being in control, being comfortable, sense of closure, affirmation/value of the dying person recognized, trust in care providers, recognition of impending death, beliefs and values honored, burden minimized, relationships optimized, appropriateness of death, and leaving a legacy and family care.

Antecedents of a good death are the result of a number of factors, but general agreement was that for a death to be good, the salient factor was that the "patient and/or family must have their wishes or preferences concerning the death honored" (Kehl, 2006, p. 282; see also Granda-Cameron & Houldin, 2012). Patient preference factors include their personal and social environment, such as their clinical condition (diagnosis, severity, and trajectory of illness), patient's and the family's financial situation and attendant life issues (Stewart et al., 1999, p. 95), as well as cultural values and religious beliefs. Moreover, the type of disease implicates the trajectory and severity of symptoms, often influencing the site of death. Paddy (2011) cited a number of conflicting opinions about the site of death contributing—or not—to a good death, many of them ascribing the low rate of home death as being the result of the medicalization of hospice care. Including location of death in the definition of a good death assumes that those who die elsewhere could only partially, but never fully, achieve a good death (Paddy, p. 36). The literature seems to favor death at home to be the only good death without crediting the number of complications inherent in a home death, particularly the philosophical question of how we die being as important, if not more so, than where we die. On one hand, home as the site of a good death bears a great deal of meaning to patients: home signifies meaning familiarity, comfort, and the company of family and friends (Gott et al., 2004); on the other hand, older people often would prefer not to die at home so as not to burden their families (Gott et al., 2004, p. 463).

Kehl (2006) and Granda-Cameron and Houldin (2012) agreed about the difficulty, in their literature reviews, of finding explicit discussions of the influences of consequences on the good death concept. Consequences of a good death applied to family satisfaction and a healthy bereavement, to professionals' work satisfaction, and to positive patient outcomes for health institutions (Granda-Cameron & Houldin, 2012, p. 637). A peaceful death was frequently cited as a consequence of a good death (Kehl, 2006, p. 283).

Surrogate terms are those used interchangeably with *good death*, such as appropriate death, decent death, desirable death, dying well, and quality of dying (Granda-Cameron & Houldin, 2012, p. 637). Related concepts were those that had a clear definition that differed from good death but that were used interchangeably with it, such as *needs of dying people, negotiated acceptable death, appropriate death, beautiful death, managed death, healthy death, correct death, happy death, peaceful death, dignified death, better death, tamed death, death with acceptance, gentle death, sacred death, medical death, natural death, good enough death, euthanasia, and meaningful life* (Kehl, 2006, p. 283). Contrary attributes were used to describe a bad death in contrast to good death and include: (1) not dying in the location of choice; (2) a prolonged death; (3) the patient being dependent; (4) the death being traumatic; (5) the patients suffering, such as being in pain or distress, cognitively impaired, and angry or fearful; (6) having a sense of unpreparedness; (7) having disorganized care; (8) having a knowledge of impending death; (9) being a burden to the family; (10) dying alone; and (11) being a young patient (Kehl, 2006, pp. 283–4).

Characteristics of a Bad Death

Clearly, the reverse of definitions of a good death constitute the representations of a bad death. Many researchers specifically discussed these characteristics.

Seymour et al. (2002) highlighted details of the SUPPORT study (Lynn et al., 1997), such as reporting that more than one in three patients had severe pain, even in those disease categories in which pain might not be expected; fatigue and breathlessness were common; one quarter of patients had moderate anxiety or confusion, with the most affected one-tenth of these patients being very troubled by psychological symptoms; and that most dying older people in this study were reported by their surviving relatives as not knowing they were dying.

Tan (2013, p. 2) observed that more than half of the participants associated pain with a bad death; that patients and families may fear bad dying even more than death itself; that a conflict between a physician and the surrogate of a dying patient can contribute to a bad death experience for the patient and family; and that a bad death likely involved having uncontrolled symptoms or distress, a lack of acceptance of the death, the death not being in agreement with the patient's or family's wishes, or the family being burdened.

Semino et al. (2014) noted that a bad death is described primarily in terms of conflict within families, lack of acceptance, rejection of physical and emotional support, and physical and emotional distress (p. 681).

Walter (2003) maintained that a bad death is one without autonomy, such as those with stroke or dementia, who cannot communicate his or her wishes, because the brain has deteriorated to the extent that there are no wishes left.

Seale (2004) considered that dying alone or dying far from home, or on another person's land, so that "one is in the company of strangers at best, is regarded in a wide variety of cultures as a bad way of dying" (p. 968).

Attributes of the Good Death in Asian End-of-Life Care

Since 1990, the Japanese Ministry of Health has supported establishment of Palliative Care Units (PCUs) and promoted specialized palliative care services. A team of palliative care specialists has undertaken several studies to conceptualize what constitutes a good death in Japan, in order to further the establishment of palliative care in that country. The first step was to conduct a nationwide qualitative study that explored the attributes of a good death in Japan for a total of 63 participants, including those with advanced cancer patients, their families, physicians, and nurses (Hirai et al., 2006). Then a quantitative study was conducted to investigate the same hypothesis using a large nationwide sample of the general population and bereaved family members (Miyashita et al., 2007). A third step involved developing a Good Death Inventory (GDI) as a measure for evaluating a good death from the bereaved family member's perspective (Miyashita et al., 2008).

The Japanese concepts of good death were expected to be different from those in the Western countries due to the difference in cultural backgrounds, especially family involvement in the decision-making process. The 17 categories that were found are listed below (Hirai et al., 2006) and each contained various attributes totaling 58. A quick scan of the list reveals a strong similarity to the categories identified by Steinhauser, Clipp, et al. (2000). The most common of the categories found in Western literature are starred and the first four categories that are in bold represent the most important domains of good death in Japan:

1. **Freedom from pain or physical/psychological symptoms***
2. **Having a good family relationship***
3. **Dying at one's favorite place/environment***
4. **Having a good relationship with medical staff***
5. Not being a burden to others*
6. Maintaining dignity*
7. Completion of life*
8. Maintaining a sense of control*
9. Fighting against cancer
10. Maintaining hope*
11. Not prolonging life*
12. Contributing to others*
13. Control of one's future
14. Not being aware of death
15. Appreciating others
16. Maintaining pride
17. Having faith*

(Hirai et al., 2006, Table 2, pp. 143–4)

This study also identified several unique findings not recognized in Western literature: the decision-making and autonomy criteria, listed under category 4, were not highly valued, as the Japanese prefer to entrust these aspects to the physicians, a trait called an *Omakase* Model (p. 145). The components alluding to the fighting spirit that were seldom found in the other studies were frequently found among these attributes (p. 145), important since it was regarded as a positive coping strategy. The taking of all available treatments is also associated with this last attribute and both are considered attributes of a good death. Within the Japanese cultural context, close relationships with family members and family preferences are highly respected such that categories #2 and #3 were critical concepts of good death (p. 144). In a 2012 ethnographic study of a good death among Japanese Americans, the factor of not being a burden—both physical and emotional—proved to be very important (Hattori & Ishida, 2012; see also Wong-kim & Burke, 2013): adequate preparation for their old age life and for their death was felt to alleviate burdens on the survivors and gave immense relief and satisfaction to them (p. 491). Another category, #16, maintaining pride, indicates that the emotional distance of the relationship with others is influenced by the Japanese cultural tendency (p. 492).

The 2007 quantitative study conducted by Miyashita et al. revealed 18 components that were very similar to the 2006 list, quantified the relative importance of each good death component in Japanese cancer care, and proved to be concepts of a good death. These findings also point to the need to incorporate challenging psycho-existential issues (p. 1094). Two major differences in quantitative results from the Western literature showed up: firstly, whereas the United States is a religious country, the Japanese have no specific religion that showed significant results. The Japanese do not want to know the serious nature of their illness, and this correlates with the category of unawareness of death as being a significant component of the Japanese style of death: dying as one sleeps, *pokkuri* and *omakase* (p. 1096).

This team also developed a measure of the good death correlates, the GDI (Good Death Inventory), which was validated to evaluate end-of-life care from the perspective of Japanese bereaved family members (Miyashita et al., 2008). In 2009, the team performed a study with the GDI in which death in the PCU was described as a good death for four of the ten aspects of a good death validated by the GDI in 2007. The PCUs were found to provide the inpatient dying individuals with whole person care. Also the team found that life prolongation treatment and aggressive treatment such as chemotherapy in the last two weeks were barriers to attainment of a good death, while appropriate use of opioid medicines were seen to promote a good death (Miyashita et al., 2008, p. 617).

A 2014 study identified the important preferences of most Chinese people for a good death and found that their attitude was similar to that of Westerners and Japanese and that the core elements of a good death were essentially the same among people of different cultural backgrounds (Haishan et al., 2014, p. 8). The attributes that were perceived as important by major respondents for a good death were maintaining hope and pleasure, good relationship with medical staff, good relationship with family, independence, environment comfort, being respected as an individual, preparation for death, physical and psychological comfort, dying in a favorite place, and not being a burden to others (p. 8). Religion and spirituality were not considered important since Chinese peoples' preference for and attitude toward death has been strongly influenced by Confucianism and Taoism. The role of the family is of fundamental importance in Chinese culture, so a dying person hopes to have emotional support from his or her family members. In traditional Chinese culture people hope to achieve a natural death and to die in their own beds. Because death has been associated with distress, fear, and mystery, Chinese people refrain from talking about death directly or openly. Physicians withhold telling bad news directly to patients, informing relatives instead.

Hong Kong Chinese patients in a palliative care service were assessed for experiencing a good death (Chan & Epstein, 2012). The authors of the study reported it as being one of the first attempts to explore the topic of good death empirically in a larger clinical sample of palliative care patients (p. 216). A more simplified method of obtaining data, Clinical Data Mining, as opposed to using more complicated existing measures, was used. The patients experiencing a good death in this palliative care service were identified from available physical and psychosocial data usually collected for clinical purposes. The aims of the study explored the proportion of good deaths achieved during the study period; determined the profile of Chinese patients who experienced a good death and the differences in their background factors, their physical and psychosocial conditions between patients who did and who did not experience a good death, and the relationship among the psychosocial factors and the patients experiencing a good death (p. 207). Among the patients included in the study, about one-fifth met the criteria, indicating the absence of pain and of patient anxiety and the presence of communication between patient and family (p. 210). Patients with a good death were older, had more children and spent more days in the palliative care service than other patients (p. 210); had a lower incidence of reported pain and better communication with family (p. 211); and experienced more fullness in life (p. 212) and less anxiety. These factors each produced notable results in achieving a good death and appeared to correlate with those found by Western researchers (Lee et al., 2012).

In Taiwan, a research group was established to define good death for Chinese terminal cancer patients in hospice care settings (Leung et al., 2009). A group of good death concepts that had previously been identified by the IOM and in prior studies by this research team were generated to assess the quality of dying, which is defined in Taiwan as indicating good death. The Good-Death Questionnaire (GDQ) developed by this team was tested on 12 attributes that were generated from 53 principles. Five meaningful factors were distilled: symptoms control, autonomy and choice, wish fulfillment, death preparation, and spiritual support that pertained to the concept of good death in the literature and our previous observations in terminal cancer patients (p. 695).

Long (2003) researched an ethnographic essay comparing the concept of good death in both Japanese and American cultures. On the issue of the cause of death, both cultures labeled death by illness categories and by non-illness categories, such as suicide, homicide, death from natural disaster. The Japanese use various modifiers of death in their speech and writing, indicating modes of death replicating the types of death set out by Lynn (2005) as well as naming them as gradual decline, sudden death, death in old age, desire to not be a burden (Long, 2003, p. 44). Regarding time, in terms of age, both cultures react in two ways: to the rapidity of death and in responding to news of serious illness or death (Long, 2003, p. 45). The other age factor is that of time in terms of rapidity. The Japanese defined the ideal death as dying suddenly, although some expressed the advantages of dying slowly as time to prepare for death. Thus, dying suddenly became a rationale for disclosing a poor prognosis only to those for whom the practical aspects of readying is deemed necessary (Long, 2003, p. 49). In the United States, people consider a sudden death as having been caused by a stroke or heart attack; the opposite extreme is considered the lingering death caused by cancer; and a sustained death by artificial means is viewed as a prolonged death. Some Americans, similar to the Japanese, voiced the desire to prepare for death by having their affairs in order. Pain was the greatest concern in both countries, while in Japan there is no distinction, as there is in the United States, between the expressions for peaceful death or mercy killing, which American bioethics dictates. Both cultures express not wanting to be a burden to others, particular if being in a vegetative state is involved. Being a vegetable was viewed by both cultures as being undesirable, particularly with regard to being a burden. In Japan, the preferred environment of death is home, viewing the technology and the equipment of hospitals as being undesirable. Many Americans also see this type of medicalization as being a bad death. A difference in meaning of going home means polar opposites: the Japanese medical system provides medical incentives for people to go home, opposed to the American system of pushing people home or to managed care or nursing facilities (Long, 2003, p. 59). In Japan, death is considered as a part of the natural process of living, considered to be natural or peaceful and a good death, as opposed to being medicalized as it is in the United States. In Japan, the dying process is a descriptive one, whereas to Americans, a good death is gained through choice and control of the dying process, a complicated issue to say the least. Strong opposition exists to being naturally alive as a human and being artificially alive, hooked up to machines and is at the root of the American belief in death with dignity, natural death, and good death. Essentially, a number of themes emerged that were common to each country: the goal of a good death is a peaceful death, the basis of which is being pain free; human suffering, both physical and mental, is embodied in the desire not to be a burden on families; a good death is accompanied by family, friends, and loved ones being present. People in both countries believe that a death should be a personalized experience, reflecting the values and life circumstances of each dying person.

Some Models of the Good Death

> . . . there is no one definition of a good death; quality end-of-life care is a dynamic process that is negotiated and renegotiated among patients, families, and health care professionals, a process moderated by individual values, knowledge, and preferences for care.
>
> (Steinhauser, Christakis, et al., 2000, p. 2481)

Can the essence of a good death be defined? According to Kearl (1996), deaths become good when they "serve not only the needs of the dying but also those of their survivors" (p. 345). Kearl stated the perspective of the survivors as: deaths are good "if the quality of life or the social status of survivors is enhanced and if their grief work is minimal" (p. 346).

Kastenbaum (2004) named five modalities of the good death: a "*good death through subtraction*" of pain and other negatives; the good death "*as a sublime and inspirational experience* through acceptance of death; *one that achieves a psychological or spiritual journey*" (pp. 122–3); is the *"continuation of a good life until it is no more"* (p. 124); and finally, the good death that *"may depend primarily on the feelings that flow back and forth between the dying person and the most treasured family and friends"* (p. 128). He suggested that one might say that we do in fact choose our own death by all the other choices we have made during our lives.

Edwin Shneidman, a psychologist, thanatologist, and acknowledged expert on suicide, outlined ten specific criteria for a good death as:

1. A *Natural* death, rather than suicide, accident or homicide.
2. A *Mature* death, after age 70.
3. An *Expected* death: Neither sudden nor unexpected.
4. An *Honorable* death produces a positive obituary.
5. A *Prepared* death: decedent arranged the necessary legalities surrounding death.
6. An *Accepted* death: Willing the obligatory; gracefully accepting the inevitable.
7. A *Civilized* death in the presence of loved one's.
8. A *Generative* death passes on the wisdom of the tribe to younger generations.
9. A *Rueful* death in order to experience the contemplative emotions.
10. A *Peaceable* death: dying scene filled with love; physical pain controlled.

(Shneidman, 2007, pp. 245–6)

Gott et al. (2008) and Walter (1994) discussed what was considered as the *revivalist* or palliative care type of good death that was prevalent in Britain. This model promised pain-free death; open acknowledgement of the imminence of death; death at home, surrounded by family and friends; an aware death in which personal conflicts and unfinished business are resolved; death as personal growth; and death according to personal preference and in a manner that resonates with the person's individuality (Clark & Hart, 2002, p. 907; Sherwen, 2014). Gott et al. (2008) claimed that the purpose behind the original palliative care philosophy was to treat those with cancer. Therefore, these researchers sought to prove that this model doesn't apply to the majority of the elderly who die of diagnoses other than cancer, often of multiple comorbidities. This population needs different parameters of care that depart from the revivalist or palliative care theory. Taking it point by point, the study revealed the differences: open acknowledgement of the imminence of death is difficult to achieve in this population since these patients have multiple comorbidities whose course of disease has no exact trajectory and are not amenable to a clinician's formulation of a prognosis. Therefore, such indeterminate prognosis promotes the patient to die an *unaware* death. Specifying a death at home, while considered more natural and desired, is not reasonable since most ill elderly are less likely to die at home due to a number of reasons (Gott et al., 2008, p. 1114). The ability to engage in personal growth when facing dying is predicated on an open awareness of death, noted above as not usual in this population. Gott et al. proposed that death facilitating personal autonomy is more acceptable in Anglophone societies and that the elderly often trust their family to make decisions for them (p. 1115). The results of this study refute most of the contentions made by Clark and Hart (2002) in benefit of the revivalist model of good death in this population of the elderly suffering from heart disease. The authors question the danger that the domination by one model of a good death, shaped by responses to cancer, has limited applicability to other groups (Gott et al., 2008, p. 1121).

In *Representations of Death*, Mary Bradbury (1999) argued that the contemporary good death concept had differentiated into three types: the ancient type of good death, which she called the *sacred good death*, has been surpassed by today's modern *medical good death*, which is being contested by the *natural death*. The contemporary sacred good death is one in which the death is seen as a social event, a time to say goodbye, which extends into the rituals that follow it (p. 148). The modern sacred death shares itself with the medical death, accepting whatever medical care is available. The medical good death is good because it is a medically controlled event that is carefully orchestrated by medical personnel, controlling the physical symptoms of dying so that the patient feels no pain and facilitating control over the timing and location of death (p. 150). Death itself is a natural event and describing any death in this way may seem logical; however, the natural death was initially a reaction to the "medicalization of death and entails retaining some sense of dignity, personhood and self-determination . . . honouring the individuality and personality of the dying person" (p. 155).

Seymour (1999) likewise positioned medical and natural deaths as polar opposites. Medical/technical interventions during dying are positioned as inhumane and unnatural with the ICU as emblematic of unnatural death (Walter, 1994). Ariès's tame death is seen as being replaced by medicalization, where death and dying are viewed as technical problems in a hospital of medical experts; where the expected picture of dying is devoid of religion and culture but replete with processes unfamiliar to lay people. Similar to Bradbury's views, Seymour cites Illich's conception of the medical nemesis, the social isolation and dehumanization of dying in hospitals that began being defined by Glaser and Strauss. The *natural death* movement promoted its view of death as a natural part of being human as opposed to being drugged to control pain, instead preferring the patient conscious and in control in order to share the dying event with family and loved ones.

Callahan (1977, pp. 33–4) also defined his concept of the ideal *natural death* as:

1. the individual event of death . . . in a life span when one's life work has been accomplished [one's vocational and professional work];

2. one's moral obligations to those for whom one has had responsibility have been discharged [particularly to one's children];
3. one's death . . . will not seem to others an offense . . . to sensibility, or tempt others to despair [its main purposes have been achieved];
4. one's process of dying is not marked by unbearable and degrading pain [pain . . . can destroy personality, sense of self, and the ability to relate to others].

The *Respectful Death* Model emerged from work at the School of Medicine at the University of Washington to establish an end-of-life (EOL) curriculum for family practice residents to benefit patients with cancer. The model supports dying patients, their families, and heath care professionals to complete the life cycle. Such an approach dictates an intimate, therapeutic, personal relationship during which personal stories are heard and incorporated into the plan of care. This method aids in the clarification of end-of-life aims and reduces conflict and suffering. Wasserman (2008) proposed this model of care for use in oncology nursing.

In an article in 1993, Callahan discussed the idea of a good death as a *peaceful* death. He questioned how technology could be made to serve a peaceful death (Callahan, 1993). He answered that instead of being viewed by medicine as an unfortunate accident, death should be established as the ultimate end point of medicine. Callahan asked why medicine did not conduct itself in a way that promotes a good and peaceful death. He maintained that the process of dying is deformed when it is subject to the violence of technological attenuation, drawn out and unduly extended by medical interventions (p. 34). Callahan defined the desired characteristics of his own good death: to find some meaning in death; to be treated with some sympathy and respect; for the death to matter to others; to not be abandoned; to not be a burden, physically and financially, to loved ones; to be conscious at the very end of life; and to have a quick death, not one with pain and suffering. He wished for the most obvious characteristic of his own peaceful death to be one that blends together the social, personal, and medical strands of his life. He believed that since medicine is unable to guarantee a peaceful death that is tranquil and pain free, the individual must summon the courage to face what does occur (p. 36).

Granda-Cameron and Houldin (2012, p. 634) defined a *peaceful death* as one that combines personal, medical, and social elements, such as finding meaning in one's own death; being treated with respect, sympathy, and dignity; hoping that one's own death matters to others; not being abandoned; not being a burden to others; being conscious and mentally intact until the very end; and hoping for a quick death with no pain or suffering.

Walters (2004, p. 408) discussed the concept of *dying with panache*, meaning to die on one's own terms and referring to a more realistic way of dying than having a good death. Elements of disapproval and uneasiness as well as expressions of anger and humor are included in the concept of dying with panache, as well as those of integrity and honesty.

Masson (2002) employed the story methodology to examine the good death concept from the point of view only of patients and their families in order to develop the multi-perspective approach to good death research (p. 193). The participants contributed experiential stories from the dying perspective, isolating three themes of reference that illustrate the complex social psychology perspective of good death: acknowledgement of tension and paradox (recognition of a fundamental tension and paradox underlying the practical realities of the context within which death and dying occurs [p. 199]); the contextualization of dying within the life lived; adoption of flexible realism, in particular concerning the site of death and pain. These three topics might today be summed up with the colloquial expression "roll with the punches", indicating that in the dying situation what you want to occur may clash with the emergent realism of the situation and needs therefore to be negotiated/renegotiated. Thus, Masson concluded that the term good death fails to convey adequately the diverse and contradictory perspectives inherent in the dying process, advocating instead the view of *good enough death* as more truthfully defining the concept.

An *aware death* was one that followed the notions set out early on by Glaser and Strauss, discussed in Chapter 1, and which Weisman also felt was necessary in his definition of appropriate death, in relation to his concept of timeliness. Goldsteen et al.'s (2006) research revealed the importance to dying people of the awareness and acceptance of impending death; of open communication about death; of taking care of one's final responsibilities; and of dealing adequately with emotions. Their conclusion highlighted the concept that what is considered a good death cannot be defined ahead of time and that each individual's requirements are personal.

Making a point similar to that of Walter (2003), McNamara (2004) wrote that no one good death exists in Britain, North America, and Australia, since social demographics, the multicultural nature of society, and institutional constraints frame the experience of dying in complex ways (p. 929). The constructions of a good death consequently became "eclectic, highly individualised or located in specific sub-cultural groups" (p. 929). McNamara maintained that the traditional hospice model of a good death therefore became inappropriate in this climate, and proposed a change in terminology to "good enough death" (p. 930; see also Sandman, 2001, p. 18). In fact, many researchers and authors have made the point that a single definition of the concept of good death does not exist.

Weisman (1972) stipulated that the purpose of studying the dying process is to learn ways of helping people attain "significant survival" so that as they near the end, they can also achieve a "purposeful death" (p. 33). Significant survival is a quality of life that intimates more than simply not dying. Purposeful death also entails more than dying: it means containing a measure of fulfillment, closure, possibly self-development, and being willing to die (p. 37). An appropriate death is a form of purposeful death.

Elements of Weisman's Psychosocial Good Death

A psychiatrist, Avery D. Weisman impressed upon his colleagues and readers that the "essence of dying extends beyond biology and is a psychosocial role as well as a physiological event" (Feifel, 1971, in Weisman, 1972, p. xi). He articulated important perspectives on the way toward better and more appropriate dying.

Weisman suspected that fear of death was at the root of most human problems, as well as their solutions. He pointed to the resurgence, in the late 20th century, of topics about death and dying, of publications and conferences concerning them, and attributed such new interest to this primary dread: death in the midst of life (1972; 1977, p. 108). Fear of dying is "an episodic state of alarm" (1972, p. 14), that is seldom fatal, a defining metaphor that expresses a condition of reality which brings together a highly personal event, imminent annihilation, with a "primitive dread that mankind has always reserved for that most ultimate event, his own death" (p. 15). Fear of death mirrors one's helplessness, a composite of fears generated by lack of meaning or motivation. Weisman cites the fear of death as a "basic concept because it seems to regard Death, capitalized to indicate its personal menace, as the embodiment of every form of human evil, failure, disgrace, disaster, and corruption" (1972, p. 16).

Discussing basic concepts and assumptions, Weisman (1972) articulates many truths about how people think about death. He cites the primary paradox as: while man recognizes that death is universal, he cannot imagine his own death—"other people die" (p. 13). He observes death as a universal phobia that man tends to believe can be avoided over and over again until it might be postponed indefinitely (p. 13). Weisman viewed denial as arising out of this paradox: that we are ill-prepared to face impending extinction and so denial must be summoned to do so.

Talking about death, the last of Weisman's basic concepts, "puts us in the role of someone who violates a taboo" (1972, p. 16). Talking about death is a painful process, so a "conspiracy of silence, denial, and dissimulation" (p. 18) arises. Talking about death entails accepting the personal reality of death as common legacy of mankind (p. 18). Acceptance of death, paired with hope, is a basic concept of Weisman's philosophy of dying and death because they insist that "mortality is a dimension of living, not merely a negation or an end-point that cancels out everything" (p. 21).

Weisman felt that any theory of death was a reflection of how humans cope, or fail to cope, with major problems of living. In this regard, he pointed to the conflict between alienation and individuality, which he viewed as linked to the inexorability of death: "We have no court of appeal. . . . Death is a property we hold in common even though most of us would gladly relinquish our claim" (p. 109). However, the following is Weisman's most telling pronouncement: "Death is whatever we choose it to be . . . to live is to strive toward a death we can live with" (1977, pp. 109–10). The problem is to find a type of death we can live with, in order to cope with the ongoing process by calling upon successful strategies from the past while correcting for differences in the present (1977, p. 114).

Since physicians are not able to predict who will die and when, and "since death is an inescapable allotment, psychosocial interventions are appropriate at almost any time, even when death is . . . remote" (Weisman, 1977, p. 115). Elements of the preterminal intervention to take toward the inexorable death are: (1) *informed consent*—a measure of the rapport presumed to exist between a patient and doctor, who are allies, not adversaries; (2) *safe conduct*— meaning that a physician is to behave with caution and prudence in guiding the patient through peril and the unknown in order to prevent dehumanization as life comes to an end; (3) *significant survival*—when the physician looks for what the patient has found significant during healthy days, something treasured in reminiscence; (4) *anticipatory grief*—a way of rehearsing death in one's own private mind that is the first phase of bereavement; (5) *timeliness*—rather than condemnation to obsolescence, timeliness of death is a highly personalized realization of completeness, in which actual survival corresponds to expected survival (1977, pp. 115–18).

The sixth psychosocial element of preterminal intervention is that for which Weisman is best known: *appropriate death*, defined as a death that a person might choose if we were able to do so, or dying in the best possible way, by surviving with "personal significance and self-esteem including minimal distress and few intractable symptoms for as long as possible" (1988, p. 67; 1977, p. 118). An appropriate death represents an absence of suffering, preservation of important relationships, an interval for anticipatory grief, relief of remaining conflicts, belief in timeliness, exercise of feasible options and activities, and consistency with physical limitations, all within the scope of one's ego ideal (Weisman, 1977, p. 119; Samarel, 1995, p. 93).

Weisman identified the four characteristic signs of an appropriate death as awareness, acceptance, propriety, and timeliness. Appropriate death is a "relative judgment, in line with reality and not idealized" (1988, p. 67); its achievement is gradual and achievable with hospice help. Achieving an appropriate death begins when the patient becomes aware that nothing more can be done and continues into acceptance of the problems inherent in the dying phase, in which caregivers attempt to carry out services that will hasten patient's/family's "acceptance of the death without removing hope" (pp. 67–8). Propriety is the third sign of a quality death and "relates to dying one's own death" (p. 69), a sort of personal bereavement involving dying as close as possible to how one wishes to die. This promotes dignity and relative autonomy in the face of the affliction, helping patients to exercise choice in where and how one dies and to participate in decisions relating to the death. Timeliness, or when one dies, too early or too late, has to do with the propriety of time of death, its expectation or relevance, being opportune but not suicidal.

These few paragraphs impart the most salient of Weisman's precepts, a wealth of wisdom borne of clinical expertise as well as education and humanity. In them, one can identify most of the concepts present in all chapters, many of them profound and true, before other researchers identified them. Many of them have become definitive of the kinds of death talked about: good enough, purposeful, appropriate, even panache, respectful, aware, peaceful.

8.3 IN CONCLUSION

> Is it possible to formulate a Golden Rule for a good death, a maxim that has the survivors in mind? I would offer . . . the following Golden Rule for the dying scene: *Do unto others as little as possible.* By which I mean that the dying person consciously try to arrange that his or her death—given the inescapable sadness of the loss-to-be—be as little pain as humanly possible to the survivors. . . . Die in a manner so that the reviews of your death speak to your better self.
>
> (Shneidman, 2007, p. 246)

Throughout this book, discussion has centered on defining and characterizing the international concepts of a good death and of psychosocial interventions to improve end-of-life care that contribute to dying well, globally. Viewpoints of physicians, staff members, caregivers, families, and patients have been highlighted, and the differences and similarities amongst these groups have been compared to one another. Elimination of pain and suffering in all dimensions (physical, spiritual, psychological, and social) assumes the top place on most lists enumerating a good death. Equally relevant named characteristics are to not prolong death artificially, timeliness of death, affording the patient autonomy and control over death, death with dignity, sudden death, dying in one's sleep, a death with a positive effect on the surviving loved ones, spiritual closure, awareness and acceptance of death, dying at home amongst loved ones/dying in an institution without loved ones present, a good relationship with medical staff, not being a burden to family, having financial affairs in order, and the sense of a life well lived (Aleksandrova-Yankulovska and ten Have, 2013; Steinhauser, Clipp, et al., 2000; Teno et al., 2001; Tong et al., 2003; Payne et al., 1996; Patrick et al., 2001; Singer et al., 1999; De Jong & Clarke, 2009). Globally, the preferences and priorities of patients, families, and clinical staff that characterize a good death are fairly similar.

In the developed world, the 20th century witnessed an increase in life expectancy due to prodigious advances in nutrition, hygiene, and the prevention of infectious diseases. The development of antibiotics and then biomedical technology has enabled ever-increasing numbers of people to avoid disease and increase their life spans. A virtual armament of medical technology harnesses chronic diseases such as cancer and the degenerative diseases that have arisen in order to prolong lives—until it no longer can.

We forget that, as Morgan remarked, "Death is still one per customer, and one for every customer" (in Wass & Niemeyer, 1995, p. 25). We trade the dread of death for the desired end to a useless and often distressing period of too-prolonged living. Pain must be relieved with well-titrated drugs, but ought fatal illness that reaches its inevitable end be extended by drug therapy, blood transfusion, surgical intervention and life support—because we can? Why equate life with good and death with evil? How is this good death?

How did all these qualifications arise and assume importance? What is the "meaning and place of death in human life" and the kind of care that is desirable at the end of life (Callahan, 2005, p. S5)? What is our stance on death? Callahan observed Ariès's tamed death that persisted unchanged for thousands of years, characterized by "practices at the end of life that stressed death's public impact" (p. 5), an acceptance of nature and destiny, and blending of death's meaning with how people died. This long era ended sometime in the middle of the 20th century when postwar medical progress was bolstered by the discovery of lifesaving drugs and biotechnologies. Now that medicine could finally "do something about death" (p. 5), physicians began the battle to save lives. The quality of life or the pain induced by these new technologies became irrelevant in the rush to battle against diseases: death was to be eliminated instead of being accepted. The divide occurred when the medical drive to research encountered the backlash against the pain and suffering it caused. The psychosocial imperatives of palliative care and death with dignity ushered in the tempering effects of comfort care and advance care planning. However, most individuals remained unwilling to address the reality of their own eventual deaths.

The principal aim of Cicely Saunders and her colleagues was to make the experience of dying better, the biopsychosocial-spiritual aspect. At that time, the meaning of a good death was a death free from physical pain, but also included the ideal of eliminating discomfort in psychological, emotional, spiritual, and social symptoms, with the ideal of dignity included. Prior to the era of medical science and technology, the idea of a good death was religious in nature: dying at peace with God. With the ascendance of biotechnology, medicine began to cure disease and its inability to do so was regarded as a failure of medicine. The ideal of a good death was seen as one that occurs in a remote, invisible future, away from home, removed to hospitals; and finally, the wished-for ideal of dying suddenly or in one's sleep, defined death as being unnoticeable. Beginning in the 1970s and by the advent of the 21st century, the taboo of talking about death morphed into a conversation enabled by the control provided by medical science: one could control the circumstances and timing of death and thereby orchestrate the desired good death (Walter, 2003; Clark, 2003; Walters, 2004; Goldsteen et al., 2006).

Kellehear (2014–15) proposed the sociological factors that contributed to the evolving meaning and place of death, citing the "complex relationship between socioeconomic position and the rise of the public health move-ment" (p. 46). Seemingly referring back to the era of the tamed death, Kelle-hear contrasted the ways in which the ruling upper classes lived with those of commoners, peasants, and the working class. Rather than the promise of comfort offered by the hospice philosophy, the working class began to aspire to the modern concept of gentrification and its idealization of "the professional and managed support of dying" of the higher social classes. The ideas of this 20th-century "public health" created the opportunity for longevity, quality of life, and professional services for everyone. The growth of the cities, industry, and the middle classes provided the atmosphere in which people sought to enjoy their increasing leisure time with as little dis-ability as possible. Kellehear maintained that these phenomena helped pave the way for the establishment of palliative care that emphasized providing healthcare via "prevention, harm reduction and early intervention" (p. 49). The concept of "the good death" arose from the positive alternative phi-losophy of palliative care that addressed dying, death, and bereavement. In the 1960s–70s, the battle began to be waged against horrible deaths from cancers—as if there were no other afflictions—and the concept of the "bad death" arose, while the concept of the meaning and place of death in society began to be entertained.

A lifestyle approach to health bolstered the pursuit of well-being and the search for a good death. The meaning of aging successfully and of how to die well has begun to enter public and private conversations. Discussions of treatment preferences, psychosocial interventions, and desires for end-of-life care center on the important bioethics of autonomy and control. People seek to control the manner of their deaths, but the length and quality of one's life are not medical or scientific matters, hence not always controllable. Internal control in a spiritual sense can replace attempts at external controls. Per-sonal history has an end point and the prospect of ending one's history pres-ents an enormous challenge: ". . . all illness smells of death, mortality, and finitude" (Sulmasy, 2009, in Schenck & Roscoe, 2009, p. 64). The tools of religion and spirituality lend significance to the search for a good death and are "essential in understanding the meaning of the aging process, suffering, disease, finitude, and dying" (p. 62).

Many people seek to prolong the death of their loved ones, despite not only the prodigious price of such longevity but also the human price of it. Rather than the inevitable end of biological human life, dying has become a "series of difficult decisions for patients and their families to nav-igate . . . opportunities to reflect on the spiritual aspects of life's end have been eroded in the process" (Schenck & Roscoe, 2009, p. 61). Families, loved ones, and caregivers become bogged down in ethical decision mak-ing, medical futility, and pain and suffering instead of soothing themselves with spiritual thoughts, awareness and acceptance, and comfort care. The touchstone of a good death and of dying well is "end-of-life medical treat-ment that minimizes avoidable pain and that matches patients' and family members' preferences" (Carr, 2003, p. 215). Likewise, a good death also embraces psychosocial-spiritual elements of social, psychological, and philosophical concepts such as maintaining close relationships with loved ones during the final days, accepting one's impending death, dying at the end of a long and fulfilling life, and not feeling like a burden to loved ones (Carr, 2003, p. 215). Many interventions to promote end-of-life care and the search for a good death have been identified and tested by clinical researchers; they are potential psychosocial-spiritual tools to use in this quest, but are they in fact implemented or is funding for it funneled instead to the medical imperative? What exactly are the barriers to the delivery of psychosocial care?

Of course, there are no good answers to these questions: what is a good death for one person may be a bad death for another. Another paradox: technology that saves lives but ruins dying (Callahan, 1993). Instead of a period of some suffering and pain, at the point when patients and families opt for prolonging life, they opt to expose their loved ones to long periods of unconsciousness, debility, and frailty: they opt for human medical intervention and technologies rather than humane treatment. The potential of humane treatment, of caring rather than curing, of spiritual peace and well-being seem to be difficult choices to make.

In a keynote address to the Institute of Medicine's National Action Conference meeting (March 20, 2015, Washington, D.C.), Atul Gawande made a number of salient points regarding end-of-life care: that well-being is more important than curing; that physicians know their patients' goals at the end of life and promote their quality of life as opposed to their survival; that people demand a life worth living in all phases of life, including its end; that doctors reject disease-focused care for goal-centered care, entailing less care which also engenders less cost and more time alive.

The meaning and place of death in modern society appears to be that which is consonant with the values, virtues, choices, beliefs, and decisions that have informed one's life in its totality. Frankl (1984, p. 168) questioned, "doesn't the final meaning of life, too, reveal itself, if at all, only at its ending, on the verge of death?" The meaning of a good death is whatever one desires it to be.

CITATIONS: CHAPTER 8

Aleksandrova-Yankulovska, S., & ten Have, H. (2013). Survey of staff and family members of patients in Bulgarian hospices on the concept of "Good Death." *The American Journal of Hospice & Palliative Care*, OnlineFirst, 1–7. http://doi.org/10.1177/1049909113516185.
Balducci, L. (2012). Death and dying: What the patient wants. *Annals of Oncology*, 23 (Suppl. 3), iii56–iii61. http://doi.org/10.1093/annonc/mds089.
Block, S. (2001). Psychological considerations, growth, and transcendence at the end of life: The art of the possible. *JAMA: The Journal of the American Medical Association*, 285(22), 2898–2906. Retrieved from www.ncbi.nlm.nih.gov/pubmed/11743842.

Bradbury, M. (1999). *Representations of death: A social psychological perspective.* London & New York: Routledge.

Breitbart, W., & Rosenfeld, B. D. (1999). Physician-assisted suicide: The influence of psychosocial issues. *Cancer Control, 6*(2), 146–161.

Breitbart, W., Rosenfeld, B. D., & Passik, S. D. (1996). Interest in physician-assisted suicide among ambulatory HIV-infected patients. *American Journal of Psychiatry, 153*(2), 238–242.

Broom, A., & Cavenagh, J. (2010). Masculinity, moralities and being cared for: An exploration of experiences of living and dying in a hospice. *Social Science & Medicine (1982), 71*(5), 869–876. http://doi.org/10.1016/j.socscimed.2010.05.026.

Byock, I. (1996). The nature of suffering and the nature of opportunity at the end of life. *Clinics in Geriatric Medicine, 12*(2), 237–252.

Byock, I. (2002). The meaning and value of death. *Journal of Palliative Medicine, 5*(2), 279–289.

Callahan, D. (1977). On defining a "natural death." *The Hastings Center Report, 7*(3), 32–37.

Callahan, D. (1993). Pursuing a peaceful death. *The Hastings Center Report, 23*(4), 33–38.

Callahan, D. (2005). *Death: The "distinguished thing". Improving end of life care: Why has it been so difficult?* Special Report 35, no. 6, S5–S8. Retrieved from www.ncbi.nlm.nih.gov/pubmed/16468248.

Carr, D. (2003). A "good death" for whom? Quality of spouse's death and psychological distress among older widowed persons. *Journal of Health and Social Behavior, 44*(2), 215–232. http://doi.org/10.2307/1519809.

Chan, W.C.H., & Epstein, I. (2012). Researching "good death" in a Hong Kong palliative care program: A clinical data-mining study. *OMEGA—Journal of Death and Dying, 64*(3), 203–222. http://doi.org/10.2190/OM.64.3.b.

Chochinov, H. M., McClement, S. E., Hack, T. F., McKeen, N. A., Rach, A. M., Gagnon, P., . . . Taylor-Brown, J. (2013). Health care provider communication: An empirical model of therapeutic effectiveness. *Cancer, 119*(9), 1706–1713. http://doi.org/10.1002/cncr.27949.

Chochinov, H. M., Wilson, K. G., Enns, M., & Lander, S. (1998). Depression, hopelessness, and suicidal ideation in the terminally ill. *Psychosomatics, 39*(4), 366–370. http://doi.org/10.1016/S0033-3182(98)71325-8.

Christakis, N. (2007). The social origins of dignity in medical care at the end of life. In J. Malpas & N. Lickiss (Eds.), *Perspectives on human dignity: A conversation* (ebook, Vol. 284) (pp. 199–207). Dordrecht: Springer.

Clark, D., & Hart, D. (2002). Between hope and acceptance: The medicalisation of dying. *BMJ, 324*(7342), 905–907.

Clark, J. (2003). Patient centred death. *BMJ (Clinical Research Ed.), 327*(7408), 174–175. http://doi.org/10.1136/bmj.327.7408.174.

Coombs, M., & Long, T. (2008). Managing a good death in critical care: Can health policy help? *Nursing in Critical Care, 13*(4), 208–214. http://doi.org/10.1111/j.1478-5153.2008.00280.x.

Costello, J. (2006). Dying well: Nurses' experiences of "good and bad" deaths in hospital. *Journal of Advanced Nursing, 54*(5), 594–601. http://doi.org/10.1111/j.1365-2648.2006.03867.x.

Coward, D. D., & Reed, P. (1996). Self-transcendence: A resource for healing at the end of life. *Issues in Mental Health Nursing, 17*, 275–288.

De Jong, J. D., & Clarke, L. C. (2009). What is a good death? Stories from palliative care. *Journal of Palliative Care, 25*(1), 61–67.

DelVecchio Good, M. J., Gadmer, N. M., Ruopp, P., Lakoma, M., Sullivan, A. M., Redinbaugh, E., . . . Block, S. D. (2004). Narrative nuances on good and bad deaths: Internists' tales from high-technology work places. *Social Science & Medicine, 58*(5), 939–953. http://doi.org/10.1016/j.socscimed.2003.10.043.

Deschepper, R., Distelmans, W., & Bilsen, J. (2014). Requests for euthanasia/ physician-assisted suicide on the basis of mental suffering—Vulnerable patients or vulnerable physicians? *JAMA Psychiatry, 71*(6), 2014–2015. http://doi. org/10.1001/jamapsychiatry.2014.185.Conflict.

Emanuel, E. J., Daniels, E. R., Fairclough, D. L., & Clarridge, B. R. (1998). The practice of euthanasia and physician-assisted suicide in the United States adherence to proposed safeguards and effects on physicians. *JAMA: The Journal of the American Medical Association, 280*(6), 507–513.

Emanuel, E. J., & Emanuel, L. L. (1998). The promise of a good death. *Lancet, 351* (Suppl. II), SII21–SII29. Retrieved from www.ncbi.nlm.nih.gov/pubmed/9606363.

Emanuel E. J., & Fairclough, D. L. (1996). Euthanasia and physician-assisted suicide: Attitudes and experiences of oncology patients. *Lancet, 347*(9018), 1805–1810.

Frankl, V. E. (1984). *Man's search for meaning* (third ed.). New York: Pocket Books.

Gibson, M. C., Gutmanis, I., Clarke, H., Wiltshire, D., Feron, A., & Gorman, E. (2008). Staff opinions about the components of a good death in long-term care. *International Journal of Palliative Nursing, 14*(8), 374–381. Retrieved from www.ncbi.nlm.nih.gov/pubmed/19023953.

Goldsteen, M., Houtepen, R., Proot, I. M., Abu-saad, H. H., Spreeuwenberg, C., & Widdershoven, G. (2006). What is a good death ? Terminally ill patients dealing with normative expectations around death and dying. *Patient Education and Counseling, 64*(1–3), 378–386. http://doi.org/10.1016/j.pec.2006.04.008.

Gott, M., Seymour, J., Bellamy, G., Clark, D., & Ahmedzai, S. (2004). Older people's views about home as a place of care at the end of life. *Palliative Medicine, 18*(5), 460–467.

Gott, M., Small, N., Barnes, S., Payne, S., & Seamark, D. (2008). Older people's views of a good death in heart failure: Implications for palliative care provision. *Social Science & Medicine, 67*(7), 1113–1121. http://doi.org/10.1016/j. socscimed.2008.05.024.

Granda-Cameron, C., & Houldin, A. (2012). Concept analysis of good death in terminally ill patients. *The American Journal of Hospice & Palliative Care, 29*(8), 632–639. http://doi.org/10.1177/1049909111434976.

Griggs, C. (2010). Community nurses' perceptions of a good death: A qualitative exploratory study. *International Journal of Palliative Nursing, 16*(3), 140–149. Retrieved from www.ncbi.nlm.nih.gov/pubmed/20357707.

Haishan, H., Hongjuan, L., Tieying, Z., & Xuemei, P. (2014). Preference of Chinese general public and healthcare providers for a good death. *Nursing Ethics, 22*(2), 217–227. http://doi.org/10.1177/0969733014524760.

Hart, B., Sainsbury, P., & Short, S. (1998). Whose dying? A sociological critique of the "good death." *Mortality, 3*(1), 65–77. http://doi.org/10.1080/713685884.

Hattori, K., & Ishida, D. N. (2012). Ethnographic study of a good death among elderly Japanese Americans. *Nursing & Health Sciences, 14*(4), 488–494. http:// doi.org/10.1111/j.1442-2018.2012.00725.x.

Hendry, M., Pasterfield, D., Lewis, R., Carter, B., Hodgson, D., & Wilkinson, C. (2013). Why do we want the right to die? A systematic review of the international literature on the views of patients, carers and the public on assisted dying. *Palliative Medicine, 27*(1), 13–26. http://doi.org/10.1177/0269216312463623.

Hirai, K., Miyashita, M., Morita, T., Sanjo, M., & Uchitomi, Y. (2006). Good death in Japanese cancer care: A qualitative study. *Journal of Pain and Symptom Management, 31*(2), 140–147. http://doi.org/10.1016/j.jpainsymman.2005.06.012.

Hopkinson, J., & Hallett, C. (2002). Good death? An exploration of newly qualified nurses' understanding of good death. *International Journal of Nursing Studies, 8*(11), 532–539.

Hughes, T., Schumacher, M., Jacobs-Lawson, J. M., & Arnold, S. (2008). Confronting death: Perceptions of a good death in adults with lung cancer. *The*

American Journal of Hospice & Palliative Care, 25(1), 39–44. http://doi.org/10.1177/1049909107307377.

Kastenbaum, R. (2004). *The final passage through life and death—On our way.* Berkeley, CA & Los Angeles, CA: University of California Press.

Kearl, M. C. (1996). Dying well: The unspoken dimension of aging well. *American Behavioral Scientist, 39*(3), 336–360. http://doi.org/10.1177/0002764296039003009.

Kehl, K. A. (2006). Moving toward peace: An analysis of the concept of a good death. *The American Journal of Hospice & Palliative Care, 23*(4), 277–286. http://doi.org/10.1177/1049909106290380.

Kellehear, A. (2014–15). Is "healthy dying" a paradox? Revisiting an early Kastenbaum. *OMEGA—Journal of Death and Dying, 70*(1), 43–55.

Lee, G. L., Woo, I.M.H., & Goh, C. (2012). Understanding the concept of a "good death" among bereaved family caregivers of cancer patients in Singapore. *Palliative & Supportive Care,* 1–10. http://doi.org/10.1017/S1478951511000691.

Lester, D. (2006). Can suicide be a good death? *Death Studies, 30*(6), 511–527. http://doi.org/10.1080/07481180600742509.

Leung, K.-K., Liu, W.-J., Cheng, S.-Y., Chiu, T.-Y., & Chen, C.-Y. (2009). What do laypersons consider as a good death. *Supportive Care in Cancer: Official Journal of the Multinational Association of Supportive Care in Cancer, 17*(6), 691–699. http://doi.org/10.1007/s00520-008-0530-1.

Lloyd-Williams, M., Kennedy, V., Sixsmith, A., & Sixsmith, J. (2007). The end of life: A qualitative study of the perceptions of people over the age of 80 on issues surrounding death and dying. *Journal of Pain and Symptom Management, 34*(1), 60–66. http://doi.org/10.1016/j.jpainsymman.2006.09.028.

Loggers, E.T., Starks, H., Shannon-Dudley, M., Back, A.L., Appelbaum, F.R., & Stewart, F.M. (2013). Implementing a Death with Dignity program at a comprehensive cancer center. *The New England Journal of Medicine, 368*(15), 1417–1424. http://doi.org/10.1056/NEJMsa1213398.

Long, S.O. (2003). Becoming a cucumber: Culture, nature, and the good death. *Journal of Japanese Studies, 29*(1), 33–68.

Low, J.T., & Payne, S. (1996). The good and bad death perceptions of health professionals working in palliative care. *European Journal of Cancer Care, 5*(4), 237–241. Retrieved from www.ncbi.nlm.nih.gov/pubmed/9117068.

Lynn, J. (2005). Living long in fragile health: The new demographics shape end of life care. *The Hastings Center Report, Spec No.* (December), S14–S18. Retrieved from www.ncbi.nlm.nih.gov/pubmed/16468250.

Lynn, J., Teno, J.M., Phillips, R.S., Wu, A.W., Desbiens, N., Harrold, J., . . . Investigators, S. (1997). Perceptions by family members of the dying experience of older and seriously ill patients. *Annals of Internal Medicine, 126*(2), 97–106.

Mack, J.W., Weeks, J.C., Wright, A.A., Block, S.D., & Prigerson, H.G. (2010). End-of-life discussions, goal attainment, and distress at the end of life: Predictors and outcomes of receipt of care consistent with preferences. *Journal of Clinical Oncology: Official Journal of the American Society of Clinical Oncology, 28*(7), 1203–1208. http://doi.org/10.1200/JCO.2009.25.4672.

Masson, J.D. (2002). Non-professional perceptions of "good death": A study of the views of hospice care patients and relatives of deceased hospice care patients. *Mortality, 7*(2), 191–209. http://doi.org/10.1080/1357627022013629.

McNamara, B. (2004). Good enough death: Autonomy and choice in Australian palliative care. *Social Science & Medicine, 58*(5), 929–938. http://doi.org/10.1016/j.socscimed.2003.10.042.

McNamara, B., Waddell, C., & Colvin, M. (1995). Threats to the good death: The cultural context of stress and coping among hospice nurses. *Sociology of Health and Illness, 17*(2), 222–244.

Meier, D. E., Emmons, C., Wallenstein, S., Quill, T., Morrison, R. S., Cassell, C. (1998). A national survey of physician-assisted suicide and euthanasia. *New England Journal of Medicine, 338*, 1193–1201.

Miyashita, M., Morita, T., Sato, K., Hirai, K., Shima, Y., & Uchitomi, Y. (2008). Factors contributing to evaluation of a good death from the bereaved family member's perspective, *Psycho-Oncology, 620*(November), 612–620. http://doi.org/10.1002/pon.

Miyashita, M., Sanjo, M., Morita, T., Hirai, K., & Uchitomi, Y. (2007). Good death in cancer care: A nationwide quantitative study. *Annals of Oncology: Official Journal of the European Society for Medical Oncology/ESMO, 18*(6), 1090–1097. http://doi.org/10.1093/annonc/mdm068.

Morgan, J. D. (1995). Living our dying and our grieving: Historical and cultural attitudes. In H. Wass & R. A. Neimeyer (Eds.), *Dying: Facing the facts* (third ed.) (pp. 25–46). Washington, DC: Taylor & Francis.

Paddy, M. (2011). Influence of location on a good death. *Nursing Standard, 26*(1), 33–36. http://doi.org/10.7748/ns2011.09.26.1.33.c8693.

Patrick, D. L., Engelberg, R. A., & Curtis, J. R. (2001). Evaluating the quality of dying and death. *Journal of Pain and Symptom Management, 22*(3), 717–726. Retrieved from www.ncbi.nlm.nih.gov/pubmed/11532585.

Payne, S., Langley-Evans, A., & Hillier, R. (1996). Perceptions of a "good" death: A comparative study of the views of hospice staff and patients. *Palliative Medicine, 10*(4), 307–312. http://doi.org/10.1177/026921639601000406.

Pierson, C. M., Curtis, J. R., & Patrick, D. L. (2002). A good death: A qualitative study of patients with advanced AIDS. *AIDS Care, 14*(5), 587–598. http://doi.org/10.1080/0954012021000005416.

Proulx, K., & Jacelon, C. (2004). Dying with dignity: The good patient versus the good death. *American Journal of Hospice and Palliative Medicine, 21*(2), 116–120. http://doi.org/10.1177/104990910402100209.

Rietjens, J. A. C., van der Heide, A., Onwuteaka-Philipsen, B. D., van der Maas, P. J., & van der Wal, G. (2006). Preferences of the Dutch general public for a good death and associations with attitudes towards end-of-life decision-making. *Palliative Medicine, 20*(7), 685–692. http://doi.org/10.1177/0269216306070241.

Samarel, N. (1995). The dying process. In H. Wass & R. A. Neimeyer (eds.), *Dying: Facing the facts* (third ed.) (pp. 89–116). New York & London: Taylor & Francis.

Sandman, L. (2001). *A good death: On the value of death and dying*. Gothenburg: Acta Universitatis Gothoburgensis.

Saunders, C. (1965). The last stages of life. *The American Journal of Nursing, 65*(3), 70–75.

Schenck, D. P., & Roscoe, L. A. (2009). In search of a good death. *The Journal of Medical Humanities, 30*(1), 61–72. http://doi.org/10.1007/s10912-008-9071-3.

Schroepfer, T. A. (2007). Critical events in the dying process: The potential for physical and psychosocial suffering. *Journal of Palliative Medicine, 10*(1), 136–147. http://doi.org/10.1089/jpm.2006.0157.

Seale, C. (2004). Media constructions of dying alone: A form of "bad death." *Social Science & Medicine, 58*(5), 967–974. http://doi.org/10.1016/j.socscimed.2003.10.038.

Semino, E., Demjen, Z., & Koller, V. (2014). "Good" and "bad" deaths: Narratives and professional identities in interviews with hospice managers. *Discourse Studies, 16*(5), 667–685. http://doi.org/10.1177/1461445614538566.

Seymour, J. (1999). Revisiting medicalisation and "natural" death. *Social Science and Medicine, 49*(5), 691–704. http://doi.org/10.1016/S0277-9536(99)00170-7.

Seymour, J., Bellamy, G., Gott, M., Ahmedzai, S., & Clark, D. (2002). Good deaths, bad deaths: Older people's assessments of the risks and benefits of morphine and terminal sedation in end-of-life care. *Health, Risk & Society, 4*(3), 287–303. http://doi.org/10.1080/1369857021000016641.

Sherwen, E. (2014). Improving end of life care for adults. *Nursing Standard, 28*(32), 51–57. http://doi.org/10.7748/ns2014.04.28.32.51.e8562.

Shneidman, E. (2007). Criteria for a good death. *Suicide & Life-Threatening Behavior, 37*(3), 245–247. http://doi.org/10.1521/suli.2007.37.3.245.

Singer, P. A., Martin, D. K., & Kelner, M. (1999). Quality end-of-life care: Patient's perspectives. *JAMA: The Journal of the American Medical Association, 281*(2), 163–168.

Steinhauser, K. E., Christakis, N. A., Clipp, E. C., McNeilly, M., Grambow, S., Parker, J., & Tulsky, J. A. (2001). Preparing for the end of life: Preferences of patients, families, physicians, and other care providers. *Journal of Pain and Symptom Management, 22*(3), 727–737. http://doi.org/10.1016/S0885-3924(01)00334-7.

Steinhauser, K. E., Christakis, N. A., Clipp, E. C., McNeilly, M., McIntyre, L., & Tulsky, J. A. (2000). Factors considered important at the end of life by patients, family, physicians, and other care providers. *JAMA: The Journal of the American Medical Association, 284*(19), 2476–2482. http://doi.org/10.1001/jama.284.19.2476.

Steinhauser, K. E., Clipp, E. C., McNeilly, M., Christakis, N. A, McIntyre, L. M., & Tulsky, J. A. (2000). In search of a good death: Observations of patients, families, and providers. *Annals of Internal Medicine, 132*(10), 825–832. Retrieved from www.ncbi.nlm.nih.gov/pubmed/10819707.

Stewart, A. L., Teno, J., Patrick, D. L., & Lynn, J. (1999). The concept of quality of life of dying persons in the context of health care. *Journal of Pain and Symptom Management, 17*(2), 93–108. Retrieved from www.ncbi.nlm.nih.gov/pubmed/10069149.

Tan, A., & Manca, D. (2013). Finding common ground to achieve a "good death": Family physicians working with substitute decision-makers of dying patients. A qualitative grounded theory study. *BMC Family Practice, 14*(14), 1–11. http://doi.org/10.1186/1471-2296-14-14.

Teno, J. M., Field, M. J., & Byock, I. (2001). Preface: The road taken and to be traveled in improving end-of-life care. *Journal of Pain and Symptom Management, 22*(3), 713–716. Retrieved from www.ncbi.nlm.nih.gov/pubmed/11532584.

Terry, W., Olson, L. G., Wilss, L., & Boulton-Lewis, G. (2006). Experience of dying: Concerns of dying patients and of carers. *Internal Medicine Journal, 36*(6), 338–346. http://doi.org/10.1111/j.1445-5994.2006.01063.x.

Tong, E., McGraw, S. A., Dobihal, E., Baggish, R., Cherlin, E., & Bradley, E. H. (2003). What is a good death? Minority and non-minority perspectives. *Journal of Palliative Care, 19*(3), 168–175.

Vig, E. K., Davenport, N. A., & Pearlman, R. A. (2002). Good deaths, bad deaths, and preferences for the end of life: A qualitative study of geriatric outpatients. *Journal of the American Geriatrics Society, 50*(9), 1541–1548. Retrieved from www.ncbi.nlm.nih.gov/pubmed/12383152.

Walter, T. (1994). *The Revival of Death.* London: Routledge.

Walter, T. (2003). Historical and cultural variants on the good death. *BMJ Publishing Group, 327*(7408), 218–220.

Walters, G. (2004). Is there such a thing as a good death? *Palliative Medicine, 18*(5), 404–408. http://doi.org/10.1191/0269216304pm908oa.

Ward, B. J., & Tate, P. (1994). Attitudes among NHS doctors to requests for euthanasia. *BMJ (Clinical Research Ed.), 308*(6940), 1332–1334. Retrieved from www.pubmedcentral.nih.gov/articlerender.fcgi?artid=2540258&tool=pmcentrez&rendertype=abstract.

Wasserman, L. S. (2008). Respectful death: A model for end-of-life care. *Clinical Journal of Oncology Nursing, 12*(4), 621–626.

Weisman, A. D. (1972). *On dying and denying.* New York: Behavioral Publications.
Weisman, A. D. (1977). The psychiatrist and the inexorable. In H. Feifel (Ed.), *New meanings of death* (pp. 107–122). New York: McGraw Hill & Co.
Weisman, A. D. (1988). Appropriate death and the hospice program. *The Hospice Journal, 41*(1), 65–77.
Wilson, K. G., Scott, J. F., Graham, I. D., Kozak, J. F., Chater, S., Viola, R. A., . . . Curran, D. (2000). Attitudes of terminally ill patients toward euthanasia and physician-assisted suicide. *JAMA Archives of Internal Medicine, 160,* 2454–2460.
Wong-kim, E., & Burke, N. J. (2013). A passage to a good death: End of life care for Asian Americans. In G. Yoo, M-N Lei, A. Oda (Eds.), *Handbook of Asian American health* (pp. 341–350). New York: Springer. http://doi.org/10.1007/978-1-4614-2227-3

Index

Weisman: appropriate death 160, 182; concept of safe conduct 68–9; and existential plight 121–2; fear of death 2; hope 115; hospice 69; preterminal interventions of inexorable death 184; psychosocial good death 183–5; purposeful death from significant survival 182

whole person care 67, 81, 176

For Product Safety Concerns and Information please contact our EU representative GPSR@taylorandfrancis.com Taylor & Francis Verlag GmbH, Kaufingerstraße 24, 80331 München, Germany